What Doctors Fail to Tell You About

IODINE & YOUR THYROID

Robert Thompson, M.D.

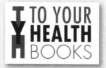

Copyright © 2015 To Your Health Books,
an imprint of Take Charge Books, Brevard, NC

Library of Congress Cataloging-in-Publication Data is on file with the Library of Congress.

ISBN: 978–0-9883866–8-6

Cover & interior: Gary A. Rosenberg • www.thebookcouple.com
Editor: Kathleen Barnes • www.takechargebooks.com

Printed in the United States of America

10   9   8   7   6   5   4   3   2   1

Contents

CHAPTER 1

We All Need It and Most of Us Don't Get Enough

Most of us have heard of iodine, but we'd be hard-pressed to recite what it does. If you're of a certain age, you probably remember your mother dabbing the yellow-brown liquid on a scraped knee and the vicious sting that followed! Maybe you remember that iodine is added to salt. Maybe you can identify iodine as a mineral. But that's probably just about it for most of us.

Before the widespread use of synthetic drugs and antibiotics, iodine was recommended for everything from healing wounds and disease, destroying bacteria and viruses, to possibly even preventing cancer.

The Nobel laureate Dr. Albert Szent-Györgyi (1893–1986), the physician who discovered vitamin C, wrote:

"When I was a medical student, iodine in the form of KI [potassium iodide] was the universal medicine. Nobody knew what it did, but it did something and did something good. We students used to sum up the situation in this little rhyme:

'If ye don't know where, what, and why,
Prescribe ye then K and I.' "

What if I told you that:

- Iodine is found in every single one of your body's trillions of cells?

- Your hormones need iodine to perform their jobs as chemical messengers in the body?

- Iodine is essential for thyroid function and every part of the cascade of metabolic processes that the thyroid governs?

- Your immune system needs iodine to function?

- It is a powerful antimicrobial that can protect you from the common cold to an infected wound (yes, Mom was right!) to cancer?

- Insufficient iodine levels lead to miscarriages?

- It is necessary for healthy breast tissue?

- Iodine is crucial for brain development in babies?

Iodine is essential to life. Without adequate stores of iodine, eventually, you may die. In the meantime, you can develop a number of diseases that negatively affect quality of life, including:

- Thyroid disease and goiter

- Breast, prostate, ovarian, thyroid, pancreatic and other cancers

- Lack of ovulation and infertility, menstrual disturbances and miscarriages

- Fibrocystic breast disease, ovarian, pancreatic and thyroid cysts, pelvic pain and possibly endometriosis

- Obesity

- Mental retardation, cretinism and possibly autism

- Allergies and asthma

- Parkinson's disease and other brain disorders

Yet approximately 2 billion people, or one-third of the world's population, live in areas defined as iodine deficient by the World Health Organization (WHO), including millions in India and China.

While WHO statistics show that about 15% of the world's population is iodine deficient, Dr. David Brownstein, author of *Iodine: Why You Need It, Why You Can't Live Without It,* says that 90% of the 5,000 patients he has tested are iodine insufficient, meaning they have just enough iodine to avoid goiter, but not enough for good health. In 1995, Dr. Brownstein writes, more than half of all pregnant women were iodine deficient. One can only assume that number is higher today.

I'll get into the wide array of health consequences of inadequate iodine intake and the bromine issue in Chapter 2, but just contemplate this one aspect of iodine insufficiency for a moment:

Iodine deficiency is the leading cause of preventable mental retardation worldwide.

What if a supplement that costs pennies a day could protect a child's brain and give him a life of promise and productivity? It's heartbreaking to think how many children are growing up right now, mentally and physically crippled, never to reach their intellectual potential, just because their mothers didn't get enough iodine during conception and pregnancy to allow their babies' brains to develop properly.

Here's a very short list of the scientifically validated health benefits of adequate iodine intake:

- Prevent breast, prostate, ovarian, thyroid and pancreatic cancer

- Maintain a healthy weight, stop food cravings and keep your metabolism high

- Boost energy and libido

- Stop "brain fog" and improve focus

- Improve dry, brittle hair and cracked skin

- Increase IQ in children, especially if given during pregnancy

- Possibly prevent autism

- Improve blood sugar control in people with diabetes

- Reduce the risk of Parkinson's and Alzheimer's diseases

What is iodine?

Iodine is a relatively rare mineral found primarily in seawater and sometimes in stones near the sea. It is also found abundantly in mountainous regions like the Himalayas, the Andes and the Alps. Low-lying land masses in Central Asia, Central Africa, much of Europe and parts of the United States around the Great Lakes are deficient in iodine.

The name for iodine comes from the Greek word *iodes*, which means violet. Iodine gas is violet colored, while solid iodine is blue-black in color and shiny.

Iodine is part of the family of chemical elements called halogens that includes bromine, fluorine and chlorine and their derivatives bromide, fluoride and chloride. Iodine is the good guy wearing the white hat, while its destructive brothers are all wearing black hats and sporting greasy mustaches, doing everything they can to stop your body from using the iodine it needs to thrive. More about toxic halogens in Chapter 2.

Iodine is present in nearly all body tissues, but it is found in the greatest concentrations in the thyroid gland, the ovaries and breasts and in the skin.

Iodine/iodide?

In nature, elemental iodine is a fairly rare mineral that is extremely caustic. We humans rarely, if ever, encounter it.

More commonly we encounter iodide, which occurs when iodine bonds with another element, most often potassium or sodium, resulting in a new compound, potassium iodide or sodium iodide. Molecular iodine is sometimes found in sea vegetables. That orangey stuff that stains your skin (in today's world, usually applied as a disinfectant before surgery) is an iodide solution.

So iodine and iodide are two sides of the same coin. Iodide is a form that the human body can tolerate, but the downside is that your body has to work a little harder to utilize the benefits of iodide.

Where do we get iodine?

Iodine is available from foods in fairly small amounts, unless you subscribe to a Japanese-style diet rich in seafood and sea vegetables.

For most Americans, food intake of iodine is not enough to produce optimal levels of iodine—or optimal health.

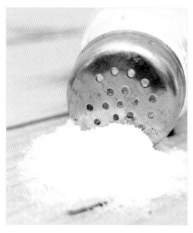

As might be expected, a large part of the Standard American Diet (SAD—and aptly named!) includes salt. I'll go into the salt dilemma at length in Chapter 2, but for now, it's important for you to know that iodized salt may contribute a small amount of iodine to your diet, but it is nowhere near what your body needs.

Then consider the toxic halogens (more in Chapter 2) that compete with iodine for "space" on the cells' receptors and block its utilization, and you'll see that we're all at risk of low iodine levels and the health problems it causes.

While we're on the subject, I'd like to point out that the American Thyroid Association says that Americans experienced a 50%

drop in urinary iodine levels in the 20 years between the early 1970s and the early 1990s. And women of reproductive age had the lowest iodine levels, barely above what would be considered iodine deficient. You'll see why that's so important to women and their babies in the coming chapters. And these figures are 20 years old. We have to guess that the levels are at least that low—and perhaps lower—now. In this same time period, thyroid cancer rates have tripled in white women since 1990.

My theory is that the time frame between the '70s and the '90s is precisely the same time frame when doctors first began advising patients to limit their salt intake. By cutting sodium, they also reduced their iodine intake, resulting in dramatically lower iodine levels.

FOOD SOURCES OF IODINE

Saltwater fish	Yogurt	Cranberries
Seaweed and sea vegetables	Cow's milk	Strawberries
	Eggs	Potatoes
Shellfish	Legumes (dried beans)	Iodized table salt
Turkey		
Cheese	Prunes	Sea salt

It's not coincidental that at this same time, food manufacturers, in another stroke of great foolishness, replaced the iodide-based dough conditioners in flours and all goods made from flour with bromide, a toxic compound that blocks iodine receptors. This was done with the blessing of the Food and Drug Administration (FDA), despite the fact that there was no research on its safety in humans. Brominated flour has been banned in many countries, some for more than 20 years. Not only is bromine used in almost all commercially produced flours in the U.S. (even organic!), it's also used on fruits and vegetables to prevent mold. Don't use any flour unless the label says, "not brominated."

It isn't salt or even sodium that is the problem. Table salt is the nutritional equivalent of white bread. It has most of its minerals removed, some of which, like potassium and magnesium, would otherwise help to balance blood pressure. Consequently, table salt causes blood pressure to fluctuate instead of stabilizing it.

The answer? Unrefined sea salt with all of the minerals we need in balance. Unfortunately, though healthier, sea salt still may not include high levels of iodine, so in most cases, supplemental iodine is required.

The government typically sets our daily requirements for nutrients ridiculously low. In the case of iodine, it's a bare 150 mcg a day for adults. Typically, we in the United States get a little more than that—about 240 mcg per day—just enough to prevent goiter (an enlarged thyroid gland indicative of iodine deficiency), but not enough for truly beneficial health effects or to overcome the bromine load to which we are all exposed.

There's nothing scary about getting more iodine in your system. After all, people in Japan consume more than 13 mg—13,000 mcg—of iodine per day just through their diet. That's 50 times more than the average American, and it hasn't hurt them a bit. In fact, it's probably contributed to better health, since we know the rates of breast and prostate cancer, fibrocystic breast disease and hypothyroidism are exceptionally low in Japan. What's more, the people of Okinawa, Japan, who consume as much as 200 mg (200,000 mcg—2,800 times the U.S. government's recommended daily intake) of iodine a day, are exceptionally long-lived.

Each clinical case is different. Everyone needs iodine, except people with untreated hyperthyroidism or a history of thyroid cancer within the last five years. However, on average, I think that almost everyone needs a supplement containing at least 12.5 mg of iodine a day. These levels are not available from today's foods grown in iodine-depleted soils. I consider a supplement containing sodium iodide, potassium iodide and molecular iodine from kelp to be the best insurance policy to provide measurable amounts of absorbable iodine.

DO *YOU* NEED IODINE? Test Yourself For Iodine Deficiency:

The following is a list of symptoms that may be experienced by someone with low or deficient iodine levels. This is *not* a diagnostic test. It is meant as a nutritional guide to raise awareness of suboptimal iodine levels. It may also help you determine whether you should have further discussions with your healthcare practitioner for clinical testing.

Please read each descriptive symptom and check off any that describe how you feel.

SYMPTOM

- ☐ I'm sensitive to cold. My hands and feet are always cold.
- ☐ In the morning my face is puffy and my eyelids are swollen.
- ☐ I put weight on easily.
- ☐ I have dry skin.
- ☐ I have trouble getting up in the morning.
- ☐ I feel more tired at rest than when I'm active.
- ☐ I'm constipated.
- ☐ My joints are stiff in the morning.
- ☐ I feel like I'm living in slow motion.
- ☐ I have foggy brain.
- ☐ The outer 1/3 of my eyebrows is missing.
- ☐ My lips are swollen and protruding, particularly the lower lip.
- ☐ I have ringing in the ears.
- ☐ My hair is coarse and falls out, it is dry, brittle, and slow growing.

- ☐ My hair is dull and lusterless.
- ☐ I have frequency of urination.
- ☐ I have impaired hearing.
- ☐ I have reduced initiative.
- ☐ My calves are big.
- ☐ My legs and ankles are swollen in the morning.
- ☐ My buttocks and thighs are too well padded and when I look in the mirror, I'm pear shaped.
- ☐ I have high blood pressure and high cholesterol.
- ☐ My heart is weak and I have a weak heartbeat.
- ☐ My stomach sags and is pushed forward by the curvature of my spine.
- ☐ My body temperature is below 97.8°F

TOTAL

RESULTS

You said Yes to **12 or more** symptoms: You would almost certainly benefit from iodine supplementation; check with your doctor to see if you have iodine or thyroid insufficiency.

You said Yes to **5 – 12** symptoms: You may want to consider testing and would be likely to benefit from iodine supplementation.

You said Yes to **0 – 5** symptoms: Although you have few symptoms you may want to consider taking iodine at a lower dosage for ongoing good health, disease prevention and detoxification.

How iodine deficiency is diagnosed

Iodine is released from the body through the urine, so the most frequently used test measures iodine in a urine sample.

The most reliable measure is an iodine loading test, which works on the premise that the less iodine you have in your body, the less will be excreted in urine when you take a large dose.

Dr. Brownstein recommends this test, in which the patient is given 50 mg of iodine and urine levels are then measured for 24 hours. Anyone with sufficient iodine should excrete about 90% of the iodine dose. Anything less means that the body is retaining iodine to make up for a deficiency. More about this in Chapter 8.

Radioactive iodine

You've probably also heard of radioactive iodine and its dangers. If you live in Southern California, you probably have potassium iodide pills on hand, distributed by the government in case of a nuclear power plant accident.

If a radiation accident releases radioactive iodine, the human thyroid absorbs it just like any other form of iodine. However, the radioactive form is highly toxic to the thyroid and can cause thyroid failure and thyroid cancer. People in the region of a radiation release are given potassium iodide to block the absorption of the radioactive iodine. If the thyroid gland is already full of all the natural iodine it needs from the potassium iodide, the radioactive iodine can't be absorbed and the thyroid is protected.

The most recent instance of a massive radiation release occurred after the Fukushima nuclear accident following the tsunami in Japan in 2011. Tens of thousands of people were exposed to high levels of radiation. It is not yet known how many people suffered thyroid damage or will suffer thyroid malfunction or cancer in the future because of that radiation release.

Radioactive iodine is also frequently used to destroy the thy-

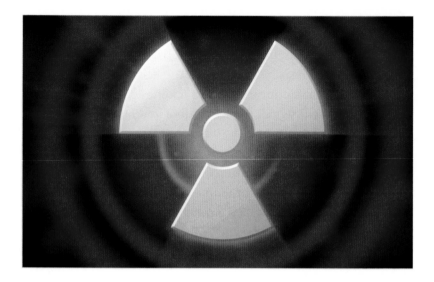

roids of people with cysts, nodules or who are deemed to be at risk for thyroid cancer.

But, as we learned in the paragraphs above regarding radiation accidents, radioactive iodine cannot destroy a thyroid that has sufficient amounts of iodine to block the absorption of the radioactive iodine. If you have enough iodine in your thyroid, it cannot be destroyed by radioactive iodine. By prescribing radioactive iodine treatment, doctors are acknowledging that they can only do this because their patients are iodine deficient. Since iodine shortfalls are known to be associated with the development of thyroid nodules and increase thyroid cancer risk, rather than destroy the thyroid, why not just take iodine?

As we progress through this book together, we'll learn more about the importance of iodine and how almost all of us can use it to create a better, stronger, healthier and happier life when iodine levels are correct.

CHAPTER 2

When Things Go Wrong

Americans are experiencing a dramatic drop in iodine levels and a corresponding deterioration in our collective health. Between the early 1970s and the early 1990s, we experienced an average drop in iodine levels of 50%. In just 20 years! That's shocking and sobering.

What's more, Dr. David Brownstein, author of *Iodine: Why You Need It, Why You Can't Live Without It*, says that about 90% of us lack sufficient iodine for optimal health, according to his tests on more than 5,000 patients. This has also been my experience in the patients I have had tested.

The low iodine blues

So what happens when your iodine levels are too low?

Thyroid disease: Low thyroid function (hypothyroidism) is often the most obvious sign of low iodine intake. Conversely, low iodine levels can also cause autoimmune thyroid disease, including Hashimoto's and Graves' diseases, which can trigger *excessive* thyroid function, called hyperthyroidism. We'll examine the symptoms of hypothyroidism and other thyroid disorders in Chapter 3, but for now, it's important to know that people with hypothyroidism may be fatigued, overweight, cold intolerant, depressed and have dry skin and hair. Low thyroid function causes all of the body's processes to slow down. Thyroid hormones are responsible for metabolic rate, energy production and brain function and development.

Breast, prostate, ovarian, thyroid and other cancers: Iodine has been validated as an anticancer agent. It works primarily by interrupting the lifespan of the wildly dividing cancer cells and protects against both hormonally related and non-hormonal cancers.

Breast disease: The link between iodine and healthy breasts was recognized as far back as 1977. Low iodine levels have been associated with fibrocystic breast disease, as well as lack of ovulation, menstrual irregularities, and infertility. Breast tenderness almost always disappears with increased iodine intake.

Obesity: Possibly related to hypothyroidism, the health risks of obesity are well known, ranging from increased risk of diabetes, heart disease and certain types of cancer. Numerous studies show the link between iodine deficiency and obesity, especially in children.

Mental retardation: Infants born with iodine deficiency are at extremely high risk of mental retardation and cretinism (stunted physical and mental development). This may also increase their risk of developing autism.

Infertility, menstrual disturbances and miscarriages: Hypothyroidism and low iodine levels are connected to infertility and a wide variety of reproductive disorders, including irregular menstruation, low sex drive, failure to ovulate, miscarriages and, in women with autoimmune forms of hypothyroidism, stillbirth.

Parkinson's disease and other brain disorders: A variety of neurological disorders, including Parkinson's and Alzheimer's disease have been connected with low iodine levels, perhaps related to the need for iodine to manufacture certain brain chemicals called neurotransmitters.

Allergies and asthma: People with low iodine levels have thicker bronchial secretions and more risk of asthma and allergies.

Inability to sweat and risk of heat stroke: Since 20% of the body's iodine stores are located in the skin, low iodine levels impair the body's ability to sweat. When you can't sweat, you get overheated and risk a heatstroke.

Our national iodine deficiency has become quite alarming. Some have even called it an epidemic. We know that things are going very wrong since iodine seems to be unavailable in adequate amounts in our food supply. But why?

It's a complicated question. Let's take it one bite at a time.

Dirt poor

In 1936, the Senate commissioned a study to determine the mineral quality of our food. We've known since the 1930s that our soils are severely mineral depleted. This

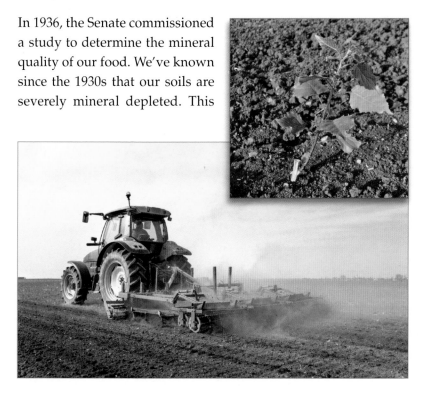

includes iodine. In simple terms, this means that when we grow produce, the plants cannot extract these vital nutrients from the soil—including iodine—if those nutrients aren't there in the first place.

Here are two of the most important conclusions of Senate Document 264 of the 74th Congress, 2nd Session, 1936:

1. "... 99 percent of the American people are deficient in ... minerals, and ... a marked deficiency in any one of the more important minerals actually results in disease."

2. "Laboratory tests prove that the fruits, vegetables, grains, eggs and even the milk and meats of today are not what they were a few generations ago. No man of today can eat enough fruits and vegetables to supply his system with the mineral salts he requires for perfect health. . . ."

Now just think about this for a moment: Remember that the "today" mentioned by the Senate committee was 78 years ago. Our government and the medical profession knew about this problem nearly 80 years ago, but has done nothing to rectify the problem, so the problem has gotten worse!

With today's farming practices, GMOs, RoundUp™ Ready seeds, herbicides, pesticides, fungicides and deforestation, it has been scientifically validated that we are at even greater risk today in 2014:

> We cannot get the nutrients we need,
> including iodine, from our food.

In 2004, a landmark study from the University of Texas at Austin examined nutritional data from both 1950 and 1999 for 43 different vegetables and fruits, and confirmed "reliable declines" in the amount of protein, calcium, phosphorus, iron, riboflavin (vitamin B2) and vitamin C over the past half century.

Researchers attribute this declining nutritional content to the agriculture industry's efforts to "improve traits (size, growth rate, pest resistance) rather than nutritional content."

While the UT team didn't specifically look into iodine content of foods, the National Health and Nutrition Examination Survey (NHANES) commissioned by the Centers for Disease Control and Prevention (CDC) confirms that our national iodine levels are plummeting.

Iodine deficiency in soil samples has been long documented, especially in Central Africa, Central Asia and much of Europe. The Great Lakes region of the United States was once known as the Goiter Belt because of the low soil levels of iodine and high rates of iodine deficiency.

So, if 99% of us were deficient in basic nutrients in 1936 and our iodine levels dropped by 50% in the decades between 1970 and 1994, where does that leave us? Pretty much at rock bottom.

It doesn't require a degree in biochemistry to surmise that we are in trouble nutritionally. Nor does it take a Ph.D. in microbiology to look at the list of health conditions caused by iodine and mineral insufficiency and see the obvious downturn in our collective health.

Worth its salt?

I skimmed the subject of table salt in Chapter 1. Now it's time to explore this subject more deeply.

A little painless history first: In the early 20th century, food manufacturers decided in all their wisdom (tongue firmly planted in cheek) that salt, a perfect food in its unrefined form containing every mineral needed by the human body in the exact proportions, should be composed solely of sodium and chloride. This refined salt was simply more convenient, pretty, white, easily finely ground and didn't clump in humidity. A decade or so later, recognizing a problem with the soaring incidence of goiters (a sure sign of iodine deficiency), it was decided that iodine needed to be added to table salt.

I'm not really sure why the food industry deemed that pure white salt was the way to go, but the American people bought the new product hook, line and sinker, and abandoned the pink or gray colored, unrefined, natural sea salt. I don't think the food industry thought about or understood that removing vital minerals would create serious problems downstream.

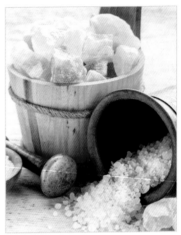

The iodized salt on your dining table probably plays little part in boosting your iodine levels, and, in any case, the iodide in salt is nowhere enough to supply your body's needs and most people don't use enough.

If you subscribe to the Standard American Diet—SAD—(I sincerely hope you don't), and you eat a great deal of processed food, you're probably getting sodium from the abundant salt and other sodium-based preservatives like sodium nitrate and sodium benzoate in these nutritional wastelands, but you're not getting any additional iodine. Most food manufacturers don't use iodized salt in what they call "food" products.

White table salt, even iodized table salt, contains iodide, sodium and chloride. But it gets worse. Contrary to popular belief, table salt is not just sodium chloride. It also contains additives that are designed to make it more free flowing. Ferrocyanide, talc and silicoaluminate are commonly added. The aluminum element in particular is problematic in a host of health problems, including Alzheimer's disease and possibly autism.

The vast majority of the healthy minerals that naturally occur in salt have been processed out of table salt, leaving it with almost no nutritional value. If you choose unrefined sea salt (easily recognized by the dark mineral flecks and usually a slightly pink or gray color), you'll be getting a small amount of *natural* iodine, as well as dozens of other minerals and trace minerals that are essential for overall health.

Dr. David Brownstein explains, "Iodized salt is a poor source of the compound iodide, because it is *not* very bioavailable for the body. Additionally, due to poor farming techniques, deficiencies of iodine and other minerals in the soil have increased. Obviously, crops grown in iodine-deficient soil will be deficient in iodine."

Health journalist Lynne Farrow, author of *The Iodine Crisis: What You Don't Know About Iodine Can Wreck Your Life*, calls this progression "the iodized salt scam."

The three-fold scam goes something like this:

1. The form of iodine that is put in salt evaporates quickly. After a container is opened, studies show it loses half its iodine in 20 to 40 days. How long does a container of salt remain in your cupboard? If you're like most of us, it may be there for years, and it will have virtually no iodine in it by the time you use it.

2. Your body can't absorb even the small amount of iodine you may be getting from table salt. We'll get to those evil halogens in a moment, but for now, it's important to understand that table salt is sodium chloride. In table salt, the chloride metabolizes to the halogen chlorine, which competes with iodine to be absorbed by your cells. In simple terms, the chlorine competes with iodine.

3. The iodine in table salt is only one form of iodine, so it doesn't do what is needed to support breast and ovarian health—and for men, prostate health. For women especially, table salt is not a good source of iodine.

White Hat and Black Hat halogens

Now is a great time to take a deeper look at the dangerous dance of halogens in our bodies.

Iodine is a halogen, like the other chemical elements, bromine, fluorine and chlorine and their derivatives bromide, fluoride and chloride.

Iodine is the only one that has health benefits for humans. It's the good guy wearing the white hat, while its destructive brothers are the bad guys in the black hats, hell-bent on blocking your body's ability to absorb and utilize the iodine that is essential to life:

- Chlorine is now almost universally used to purify municipal water supplies instead of iodine. Even if you don't drink municipal water, if you shower or bathe in it, you are exposed to its toxic effects. Perchlorate, a highly toxic chlorine derivative used for rocket fuel among other things, has become pervasive in the water supply.

- Fluoride is now found in almost all toothpastes and municipal drinking water supplies. Some unenlightened dentists still insist on fluoride treatments to prevent tooth decay, despite the fact that there is no scientific evidence that the application of this toxic waste product has any positive effects. Fluoride has been confirmed to interfere with thyroid function and has been associated with some types of cancer.

- Bromine, also known to cause cancer, replaced iodine in commercial baked goods and almost all flours more than three decades ago. You'll also find potassium bromide in soft drinks, plastics, cans and jars, many personal-care products, sprayed on fruits and vegetables to inhibit mold, especially berries, in electronics and it has also been added to some vaccinations and asthma inhaler medications to replace mercury as a preservative. There are few or no labeling requirements. It's impossible to avoid breathing bromine fumes in any house, car, school or office building, so we are all continuously exposed to this cancer-causing chemical.

Other iodine robbers

Recently, we've also learned that soy-containing foods in some circumstances may block your body's ability to use iodine, and, with the increasing epidemic of gluten sensitivity, there are signs that gluten may also block iodine absorption.

This all adds up to a conspiracy on the part of the Black Hat halogens and their partners in crime, soy and gluten, to rob your body of its ability to use iodine to complete millions of vital metabolic functions every day.

The Black Hat halogens compete with White Hat iodine for access to your cellular function. Each cell has receptors, which function just like locks. All halogens have the keys to these locks—and the Black Hats do everything they can to prevent White Hat iodine from opening the locks.

Here are a few ways to avoid bringing any more Black Hat halogens into your home and your body:

1. Avoid all products made with brominated flours. Even products made with organic flours contain bromine, since it is considered a natural substance. I know of only one brand, King Arthur Flour, which is not contaminated with bromine. Look for the words "non brominated" on the label to be sure. Bromine is also found in many soft drinks, wine and beer.

2. If you have a municipal water system, invest in a whole house water-filtration system to prevent absorption of halogens through your skin when you shower.

3. Don't use fluoridated toothpaste.

4. Avoid soy and gluten as much as possible.

5. Don't eat or drink food that is stored in plastic containers.

6. Avoid soft drinks.

7. Look for chemical-free personal-care products.

8. Ventilate your home and your workspace well. Open windows whenever weather permits.

We owe a great deal to Dr. Guy Abraham, the UCLA professor who pioneered iodine research through the Iodine Project for this information about toxic halogens and much more.

Iodine supplements

Nearly everyone needs some level of iodine supplementation and most of us need a lot of it to get to optimal iodine levels (90% excretion on a 24-hour loading test).

The good news is that iodine, the White Hat halogen, can fight back and overcome the Black Hat chlorine, fluorine and bromine molecules, crowd them off the cell receptors and be back in the game with access to your cells, if you get enough. It takes a lot of iodine to counteract and reverse the effects of bromine.

As you've seen from this chapter, it is virtually impossible to get enough iodine from food and table salt.

The answer is to find the best possible supplement, one that offers iodine in three important forms, each with its own benefits:

- Potassium iodide for thyroid health

- Sodium iodide for thyroid, prostate, pancreatic, brain and immune system health

- Molecular iodine from kelp for breast, ovarian, prostate and reproductive system health

Note: Some people are "allergic" to iodine. This almost always means they are allergic to the organic form of iodine , such as the Betadine that is used in hospitals. It is nearly impossible for a human to get too much iodine. Excess iodine is just excreted through the urine when it is not needed. There is no known toxicity for iodine except untreated cases of hyperthyroidism. For those who experience symptoms of intolerance (such as diarrhea or stomach upset), start with small doses and gradually build up to the optimal dose.

CHAPTER 3

Iodine, Thyroid Disorders, Obesity and More

The thyroid is the body's major thermostat, and keeping it operating well keeps your metabolism running at the perfect pace.

Every single cell in your body depends on the thyroid gland for hormones that instruct it how to function.

This tiny butterfly-shaped gland at the base of your throat weighs less than an ounce and secretes less than a teaspoon of thyroid hormones in an entire year, but when things go wrong with your thyroid, they go wrong everywhere in your body.

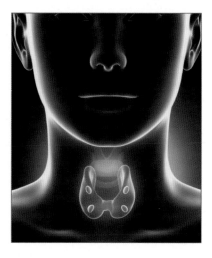

The thyroid hormones regulate metabolism, the rate at which your body converts fuel (food) into the energy you need to power everything you do, the rate at which your body uses fats and carbohydrates, controls your body temperature, heart rate, the production of protein and your body's ability to regulate the amount of calcium in your blood.

Too little, too much, just enough . . .

Too little thyroid hormone causes a disease called hypothyroidism, in simple terms, low thyroid function. In this most common of thyroid disorders, you are like a wind-up toy that is slowly winding down.

Too much thyroid hormone and the hormones flood your system, causing you to be hyper and frenzied, tachycardic (fast heart rate) and have heart palpitations, all symptoms of hyperthyroidism.

Autoimmune thyroid diseases like Graves' and Hashimoto's are another story and can actually cause you to be both hypo- and in some cases, hyper- thyroid.

The thyroid balances your body through the production of thyroid hormones. The main ones are triiodothyronine (T3) and thyroxine (T4). These hormones are synthesized from the amino acid tyrosine and the mineral iodine.

The U.S. government estimates that 4.6% of the population over the age of 12 has clinically low thyroid function. Other sources suggest a much higher rate, as high as 10%, based on the concept that at least half of the people with low thyroid function are unaware of the condition or they are undiagnosed because of the painfully cumbersome process of getting a diagnosis and treatment.

Over a lifetime, 12% of the population will develop a diagnosable thyroid condition, says the American Thyroid Association (ATA). Women are far more susceptible to hypothyroidism, especially women over 60. The ATA estimates that women have 5 to 8 times more thyroid disease than men.

Iodine inadequacy and calcium excess are the primary causes of most types of thyroid disorders. You know from earlier chapters that rates of iodine deficiency have skyrocketed in the United States and around the world.

Without iodine, the thyroid gland cannot manufacture hormones, T3 and T4. Iodine is a major part of the chemical structure of both of these thyroid hormones.

A goiter (swelling of the thyroid area as a result of impaired thyroid activity) is a sign the thyroid is producing either too little or too much thyroid hormone. Goiters are not often seen today, believes Dr. David Brownstein, author of *Overcoming Thyroid Disorders*, because iodized salt gives us just enough iodine to prevent goiters, but nowhere near enough to take care of the rest of the body's needs.

Do you have a thyroid problem?

Here's a list of symptoms of hypothyroidism. You'll see that some of them may seem contradictory and some are the same for both

SYMPTOMS OF HYPOTHYROIDISM (UNDERACTIVE THYROID)

Blood pressure high or low	Eyebrows—thinning and loss of outer third	Memory loss
Brain fog	Eyelid swelling	Menstrual irregularities
Brittle nails	Fatigue	Miscarriage, stillbirth
Carpal tunnel syndrome	Fibrocystic breast disease	Muscle cramps
Cold hands and feet	Food cravings (sweet and salt)	Muscle weakness
Cold intolerance	Hair thinning or loss	Nervousness
Constipation	Heart rate slow	Numbness in feet, hands
Depression	Heartburn	Puffy eyes
Difficulty losing weight	Heat intolerance	Slow wound healing
Difficulty swallowing	Hoarse voice	Snoring
Dry, itchy skin	Infertility	Throat pain
Elevated cholesterol	Insomnia	Tinnitus
	Irritability	Weight gain

SYMPTOMS OF HYPERTHYROIDISM (OVERACTIVE THYROID)

Blood pressure high	Hair loss	Nervousness
Diarrhea	Hand tremors	Palpitations (heart pounding)
Difficulty concentrating	Heat intolerance	
	Increased appetite	Rapid heartbeat
Eyes protruding	Itching overall	Restlessness
Fatigue	Irregular menstrual periods or absence of periods	Skin clammy
Frequent bowel movements		Skin flushing
		Sleep problems
Goiter (visibly enlarged thyroid gland)		Weakness
	Nausea and vomiting	Weight loss unexplained

hypothyroidism and hyperthyroidism, e.g. hair loss and fatigue. All or almost all of these symptoms can also be symptoms of other health problems. Having more than three or four of these symptoms should spur you to investigate your thyroid function more deeply.

What to do if you suspect you have a thyroid disorder

There is a simple do-it-yourself test that was considered the definitive diagnosis until a slew of fancy and unreliable blood tests came into fashion about 50 years ago and doctors began to interpret the test results inconsistently and without regard for signs or symptoms of the disease.

Before the TSH, T3, T4 Reverse T3 and T4 and thyroid antibody tests, there was only one simple test that gave doctors the answer. It's still in use today.

All you need is a common thermometer to conduct your own thyroid function test, based on the premise that low thyroid function causes metabolic rates to slow down and results in cooler body temperatures. Dr. Broda Barnes, a pioneer in understanding, diagnosing and treating thyroid disorders, popularized the test, which had been known for decades. The Basal Body Temperature (BBT) remains the most accurate and reliable test there is today. The BBT fell into disuse with the advent of various tests for thyroid hormones in the blood, which may or may not give accurate or complete answers.

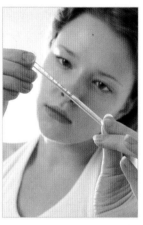

1. Keep your thermometer by your bed (digital or non-digital is OK).

2. Take your temperature when you first awaken, before you get out of bed.

3. Repeat every day for a week.

If your average basal temperature is below 97.8 degrees Fahrenheit, you most likely have hypothyroidism. It's as simple as that.

Note: *Women should not do this test around the time that they are ovulating, but choose another time of the month (preferably days 1–12) to do this test.*

Getting diagnosed with a thyroid disorder, particularly hypothyroidism, can be a long and frustrating journey, primarily because many doctors are uninformed. Some (their number is thankfully dwindling) will simply palpate the thyroid gland and pronounce that "everything is fine" if they feel no nodules.

Others will order a blood test called the thyroid stimulating hormone (TSH) test, and, if the results come back within the reference range, they tell you to get off the couch and eat less, that there's nothing wrong in spite of your numerous signs and symptoms. For more than a decade, doctors have disagreed about the "normal" ranges for TSH. Many labs and practitioners have unrealistically wide "normal" ranges that leave many people with hypothyroidism out in the cold, quite literally.

If you suspect you have hypothyroidism and your TSH test comes back "normal," insist on being tested for Total T3, Free T3, Free T4, Reverse T3 and thyroid antibodies. This will give you and your doctor much more reliable tools to determine what the thyroid is really doing or, more likely, what it's not doing. The Total/Reverse T3 ratio is also the most accurate test to insure one is on the correct treatment.

You'll be even better off if your doctor understands thyroid hormones, proper thyroid hormone replacement and its link to other conditions, including adrenal insufficiency.

Treatment for hypothyroidism

Conventional medicine usually treats low thyroid function with a synthetic form of T4 called levothyroxine (Synthroid, Levoxyl, Levothroid, Unithroid), the free-circulating thyroid hormone that must be converted to the T3 form before it becomes active. T4 is the storage form of thyroid hormone. This forces your body to work harder to get the hormone it needs. As an interesting side note: levothyroxine was the most prescribed drug in the U.S. in 2013, according to the research firm IMS Health.

Iodine supplementation may help you use the synthetic thyroid hormones better. Sometimes a doctor will prescribe liothyronine (Cytomel), a synthetic form of T3, if there is evidence the body's ability to convert T4 is impaired. I look at the TT3/RT3 ratio (normal is 10-14) to determine the correct level of T3 increase or T4 decrease needed to correct this ratio and to know for sure there is adequate T3 conversion and not too much thyroid hormone being given.

Increasingly, doctors who prefer a more natural approach prescribe thyroid hormones made from pig thyroid glands. The most widely used brands are Nature-Throid, Armour and Westhroid, which contain the full spectrum of four thyroid hormones (T1–T4), more closely mimicking human thyroid function.

A diagnosis of hypothyroidism and any prescription treatment plan will almost inevitably require a comprehensive approach, some experimentation and retesting until the correct balance is achieved.

Iodine is essential for the treatment of hypothyroidism. Without iodine, all of the thyroid hormones in the world won't help your thyroid create and convert the thyroid hormones you need or allow you to stay at the levels you need for optimal health. If you've been diagnosed with hypothyroidism, look for an integrative practitioner to partner with and consider a supplement with potassium iodide, sodium iodide and molecular iodine. Some extra L-tyrosine will help, too. When looking specifically for a thyroid product, consider at least 15 mg of the three forms of iodine, combined with 200 mg of L-tyrosine in each capsule. The starting dose many integrative practitioners recommend is two capsules each morning.

A basal body temperature above 97.8, is the best and most accurate indicator of correct thyroid function and treatment.

If you are using iodine alone, you can find excellent iodine supplements with 12.5 mg of these three iodine forms.

There has been extensive discussion of the safe levels of iodine intake. Consider this: The Japanese, with their diet high in iodine-rich seafood and sea vegetables, typically consume more than about 13 mg of iodine daily, 50 times what the typical American ingests, all without negative side effects. In fact, Japan has far lower national rates of breast and prostate cancer and hypothyroidism than are found in the Western world. Iodine dosages as high as 50 mg a day are frequently recommended for patients with hypothyroidism, cancer and other serious iodine deficiency conditions.

Lifestyle treatments for hypothyroidism

A variety of simple lifestyle adjustments can help rebalance thyroid hormones and help detoxify your body from Black Hat halogens.

Managing stress is essential to overall health. It's especially important to people with thyroid disorders because stress can cause blood sugar imbalances, food intolerances (especially to gluten), digestive dysfunction, chronic infections and inflammation, all of which tell the adrenal glands to keep pumping out stress hormones. Those stress hormones have a profound effect on the ability of the thyroid to convert T4 into usable T3, cause an increase of RT3 production and can, over time, create thyroid hormone resistance.

Lots of exercise is important for reversing the low-energy loop and making thyroid receptor sites more sensitive to thyroid hormones.

Saunas and soaks are great ways to help your body detoxify and remove the Black Hat halogens. Far-infrared saunas are excellent tools for detoxification. If you have a hot tub, please do not use bromine or chlorine as a disinfectant. There are more natural forms of disinfection like ozone purification systems and mineral cartridges that keep those Black Hat halogens out of your life. If you are taking a long, hot soak, add some Epsom salts to your bathwater for extra magnesium to help pull out toxins.

Filter your water and change your toothpaste to limit your exposure to toxic fluoride. Most municipal water systems and nearly all commercial toothpastes still contain fluorine, despite their well-documented iodine-blocking properties that impair thyroid function.

Adjust your diet to reduce foods called goitrogens. These are foods that suppress thyroid function by impairing the body's ability to use iodine. While most of the foods on this list are healthy foods, they're just not helpful for people with thyroid disorders and should be consumed in moderation in their raw state.

Top 10 Goitrogenic Foods

Bok choy	Kale	Rutabagas
Broccoli	Kohlrabi	Soy (anything)
Cabbage	Mustard and	Turnips
Cauliflower	mustard greens	

Foods with Smaller Amounts of Goitrogens

Bamboo shoots	Pears	Sweet potatoes
Millet	Pine nuts	Wheat and other
Peaches	Spinach	gluten-containing
Peanuts	Strawberries	grains

Radioactive iodine treatment for hyperthyroidism

If you are unfortunate enough to be diagnosed with hyperthyroidism, it is very likely that your doctor will want to use radioactive iodine to block the runaway production of thyroid hormones. Modern medicine conveniently forgets to tell you that this high dose radioactive iodine treatment will destroy your thyroid gland for life. It doesn't address the underlying cause of the problem, and you will need to be on thyroid hormones for as long as you live. As I mentioned in Chapter 1, radioactive iodine will not be effective in destroying the thyroid if you have sufficient iodine.

To make matters worse, the radioactive iodine will bind to other cell receptors for iodine, and it will concentrate in the places where iodine is more frequently found in the body, especially in women's breasts, increasing the risk of breast cancer. More about that in Chapter 4.

Medical science has long known that radiation and radioactive substances cause cancer, so it should come as no surprise that people who have radioactive iodine treatments for hyperthyroidism have a 400% greater risk of death from thyroid cancer *plus* an increased risk of stroke and death from other types of cancer.

Yes, hyperthyroidism is a serious health problem and it must be treated. Untreated hyperthyroidism can cause heart problems like atrial fibrillation, increasing the risk of stroke, cardiomyopathy and osteoporosis. If you are pregnant, hyperthyroidism increases the risk of preeclampsia, early labor, low birth weight babies and hyperthyroidism in the baby.

Among the underlying causes of hyperthyroidism are infection, toxicities, food allergies (gluten intolerance, for example) and nutritional imbalances. Dr. Brownstein believes that iodine is a common denominator in treating *all* of these problems. What's more, iodine is the key to treating hyperthyroidism with far fewer long-term health risks.

Thyroid and lack of iodine

So, how did your thyroid and millions of other thyroids worldwide get so far out of whack?

Take a guess.

If you answered, "Iodine deficiency," you get a gold star. You already know that the government recommended iodine intake is woefully inadequate to promote a healthy thyroid and to keep your entire body in optimal health.

You also know that our dramatic increase in exposure to toxic halogens (the Black Hat halogens chlorine, fluorine and bromine) blocks the body's ability to use the little iodine we get.

So we have an epidemic of hypothyroidism and other thyroid disorders (Graves' and Hashimoto's disease, thyroid cancer), all of which have iodine deficiency as an underlying cause.

Iodine supplements offer the most powerful means of rebalancing thyroid hormones and neutralizing toxic halogens.

Thyroid, iodine and the struggle for weight control

Science proves the following:

1. Hormones, especially thyroid and insulin, control body weight.

2. Insufficient thyroid hormone production can cause numerous health problems, not the least of which are food cravings and weight gain.

3. Insufficient iodine intake is one of the largest contributors to hypothyroidism.

So you don't have to be a research scientist to figure out that inadequate iodine stores in your body translate to excess weight.

"The healthy functioning of the thyroid is essential to maintaining metabolism and preventing the accumulation of body fat," writes Burton Goldberg in *Alternative Medicine.*

An underactive thyroid and a thyroid hormone resistant gland slows metabolism, causing dramatically fewer calories to be burned, leaving you tired, irritable and sluggish, and less likely to exercise.

In addition, in *Asian Health Secrets,* author Letha Hadady theorizes that an underactive thyroid also promotes excess weight and cellulite by causing water retention.

Iodine supplementation may also increase weight loss in the case of low thyroid function by addressing the thyroid insufficiency and raising the BMR (basal metabolic rate), effectively burning more calories.

Finally, we've known for at least 20 years that overweight women are more susceptible to breast cancer. And we know that iodine shortfalls increase the risk of breast cancer. (More about that in Chapter 4.) Early research from the University of Virginia linked iodine insufficiency, a high fat diet and breast cancer as far back as

1979. Later researchers have confirmed that excess estrogen attached to fat cells are the probable cause of the increased risk of breast cancer in overweight women.

By now, you've probably noticed that much of the research on iodine and thyroid and many other health problems is what we might call peripheral (on the side, if you will) or tangential (at an angle, not direct). You're probably wondering why there isn't more direct research on iodine, an inexpensive and highly effective means of treating and preventing many serious health problems, including obesity.

The answer is simple: There's no money in it. Trials on human subjects cost millions of dollars. Iodine is a plentiful and inexpensive mineral that is not patentable, since it is a substance occurring in nature. Translation: The big pharmaceutical companies can't make millions and billions of dollars on it like they can on prescription drugs, so they don't bother studying it.

It's their loss and your gain, since Big Pharma won't be able to charge you $100 or more per prescription or whatever nonsense it dishes out with so many prescription drugs.

But there is some research:

- A 2013 Russian study showed that overweight adults aged 30 to 65 were given a jam laced with iodine and chromium and no other dietary restrictions. Members of the group lost 5% of their body weight and reduced their waist size, blood pressure and triglyceride levels significantly more than a control group that was given standard diet advice to restrict calories and fat.

- A 2011 Turkish study showed that the urinary iodine status of obese women was directly related to body mass index and levels of leptin, a hormone found in fat cells that tells your brain you are starving and should eat more. The bottom line: with sufficient iodine intake, weight drops and there are fewer fat cells that keep telling your brain you are starving.

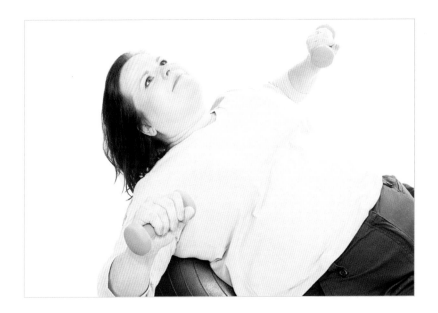

Food cravings

Sugar, salt and fatty food cravings are all signs of thyroid insufficiency, insulin resistance and mineral deficiency. By now you know that thyroid insufficiency means you're not getting enough iodine. Think of these cravings as your body's cry for help. Your body's lowered metabolism means that those extra calories, and particularly the sugar that converts to fat cells, will result in weight gain.

Carb cravings are very common among people with hypothyroidism and insulin resistance. Scientists haven't figured out exactly why this happens, but it may have something to do with the anxiety, depression and fatigue that often accompany low thyroid function and the brain's response that sparks the desire for carbs that stimulate the release of the feel-good, appetite-suppressing neurotransmitter, serotonin.

Leptin comes into play big time in the food cravings and weight gain cycle. This hormone tells you when you have had enough to eat and also triggers a fat-conserving starvation response when it thinks you haven't had enough. This is especially true for yo-yo dieters, whose leptin mechanisms get confused, they battle cravings and their bodies refuse to let go of excess fat.

Leptin's ability to tell you when you have had enough food has also been connected to the accumulation of toxic chemicals in your body, most notably chlorine, fluorine and bromine. Where have we heard of those before? Those are the Black Hat halogens that block your body's ability to use iodine, in this case, triggering food cravings, overeating, slow metabolism, weight gain and even type 2 diabetes. What a vicious circle!

CHAPTER 4

Iodine, Women and Breast Health

I'm going to make a bold statement here: *Iodine shortfalls coupled with bromine and other toxic halogens cause fibrocystic breast disease and breast cancer.*

For more than 60 years, science has confirmed that iodine concentrates in breast tissue. I've already mentioned that there is a high concentration of iodine in the thyroid gland and the ovaries.

Breast tissue contains the body's third highest concentrations of this essential mineral, so shortfalls in iodine needs have a highly negative impact on breast tissue. When you don't have enough iodine in your diet, or when you are iodine compromised because of exposure to the toxic halogens: chlorine, fluorine and bromine, the breast and thyroid compete for the little iodine that is available. The result is that the iodine supply in the thyroid and breasts is depleted, opening the door to thyroid related disorders (see Chapter 3), fibrocystic breast disease and breast cancer.

Let's take them one at a time:

Fibrocystic breasts or fibrocystic breast disease

This condition has become so common that some doctors argue it isn't a disease at all. More than half of all women experience fibrocystic breasts and cyclic breast tenderness at some point in their lives.

Women with fibrocystic breasts have bumpy, lumpy breasts that may have hardened areas. They are sometimes painful. Pain has been linked to hormone fluctuations during the menstrual cycle, caffeine intake and the use of oral contraceptives.

Ropy scar-like tissue or cysts and lumps characterize fibrocystic breast disease. Many women have both symptoms and some have nipple discharge as well. The lumps and bumps generally change throughout a woman's menstrual cycle. A lump that does not change during a menstrual cycle or on a postmenopausal woman who is not on hormone replacement may signal another problem and requires further investigation.

Most professionals agree that fibrocystic breasts do not increase your risk of breast cancer, except in women with another risk factor, such as family history of breast cancer or other genetic predispositions to the disease. Some medical practitioners argue that the lumpiness of fibrocystic breasts may make it more difficult to feel potentially cancerous lumps in a breast self-examination (BSE).

Fibrocystic breasts are usually quite dense, so they are somewhat resistant to mammograms, so many women with this condi-

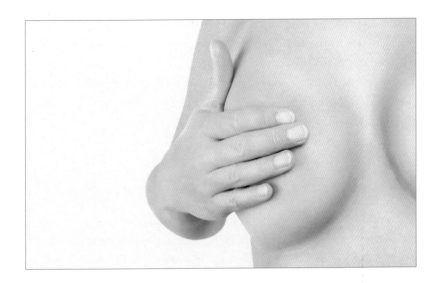

tion are referred for diagnostic ultrasounds that can more easily distinguish between healthy and diseased breast tissue.

However, there is a common thread between fibrocystic breasts and breast cancer: Both conditions are related to insufficient iodine intake and halogen toxicity.

Several studies in animals and humans give strong evidence that:

- Animals that were intentionally deprived of iodine developed fibrocystic breasts.

- Supplementation with iodine reduces the lumps, bumps and hard spots and even reduced breast size in animals. Just taking 6 mg of iodine a day for six months stopped the pain of fibrocystic breasts for half the women in a 2004 study reported in the journal *Breast*.

I am convinced that bromine's interference with iodine also contributes to endometriosis and pelvic pain.

Estrogen, iodine and breast cancer

Iodine deficiency causes estrogen production to become unbalanced and dysfunctional. At the same time, this double whammy causes breast tissue to be more sensitive to estrogen, cystic changes occur, increasing the risk of breast cancer. That's a double-barreled shotgun.

Today, **one in seven** American women will develop breast cancer during her lifetime. Compare that to 30 years ago, when iodine consumption was much higher, bromine use was much lower, and one in 20 women developed breast cancer. Women in Japan who consume high amounts of dietary iodine have much lower rates of breast cancer and thyroid problems. However, when women emigrate from Japan to the United States and begin eating a Western diet, with its fractional amount of iodine and loads of bromine exposure, their incidence of breast cancer and thyroid disease increases dramatically.

Interestingly, the 50% drop in our national iodine levels since the 1970s parallels the increase in breast cancer rates, despite the National Cancer Institute's contention that the higher rates are due to earlier diagnosis and an aging population. The drop in iodine levels and the steadily rising breast cancer rates—and what Dr. David Brownstein calls an epidemic of hormone-sensitive cancers like breast cancer—are simultaneous with the removal of iodine from refined flours and the substitution of bromine, which blocks the body's absorption and utilization of iodine. These are too many "coincidences" to be disregarded.

Another interesting noncoincidence is that the incidence and severity of breast cancer is lower in Japan and Europe than in the United States, attributed to dietary differences, the lack of bromine in refined flours and the absence of fluoride in municipal drinking water. For example, less than 1% of public drinking water is fluoridated in Japan, and virtually no European countries fluoridate their drinking water. Potassium bromate, the form of bromine routinely added to flours in the United States, is banned in the European Union, and Japanese flour manufacturers voluntarily stopped using potassium bromate in their products in 1980. One Japanese company resumed using the iodine-blocking toxic halogen in 2005, but most of Japan's flour is still bromine free. The absence of these Black Hat halogens from the lives of Japanese and European women offers powerful protection against breast cancer.

A final noncoincidence is our rising exposure to xenoestrogens —environmental estrogens present in plastics, pesticides, meat and dairy products—that trigger further estrogen imbalances.

It is impossible to ignore the weight of the evidence against the conscious addition of toxic halogens to our food supply, contaminants that have been scientifically proven time and time again to deplete iodine stores, disrupt iodine function and cause a variety of diseases, including breast cancer. I am convinced that bromine's interference with iodine also contributes to endometriosis and pelvic pain.

Dr. David Brownstein says, "Perhaps rectifying iodine deficiency will be the missing piece of the puzzle to solving the riddle of breast cancer."

He adds, "I believe all women need to be evaluated for their iodine status before they reach the stage of breast cancer."

Dr. Brownstein has documented numerous cases among his patients that demonstrate that iodine treatment reduced breast cancer tumor sizes and induced remissions with no other treatment than the use of iodine.

Let's step back for a moment and take a look at the role of estrogen and iodine in breast health or ill health.

Estrogen is a sex hormone predominant in women, produced primarily by the ovaries, with smaller amounts produced by the adrenal glands and fat tissue. Excess estrogen stored in fat tissue is considered a risk factor for breast cancer in women.

Men do produce small amounts of estrogen, about 10% of the amount found in women, mainly made by the adrenal glands, fat tissue and liver. And, by the way, men can and occasionally do get breast cancer and the incidence of breast cancer in men is rising dramatically.

Just a quick primer on human estrogen: There are three types of estrogen: estrone, estradiol and estriol. The weakest of these, estriol, stimulates breast tissues less than estrone and estradiol. In fact, there is a growing body of research that confirms that estriol protects against the cancer-causing effects of estradiol and estrone.

In an important 2002 study from the U.S. Army and performed at the Public Health Institute, Oakland, California, researchers compared estriol levels during pregnancy with the occurrence of breast cancer in the same women 40 years later. Of the 15,000 women entered in the study, those with the highest levels of estriol relative to other estrogens during pregnancy had the lowest cancer risk. In fact, women with the highest level of estriol during pregnancy had

58% lower risk for breast cancer compared with women who had the lowest estriol levels. The researchers also noted that Asian and Hispanic women had higher estriol levels compared with other racial groups, an interesting finding since Asian and Hispanic women have the lowest breast cancer rates.

The researchers concluded, "If confirmed, these results could lead to breast cancer prevention or treatment regimens that seek to block estradiol estrogen action using estriol, similar to treatment based on the synthetic anti-estrogen tamoxifen."

So where does iodine come into this equation? Research from Jonathan Wright, M.D., a bioidentical hormone therapy pioneer, shows that iodine helps maintain the correct balance of the three types of estrogen and even to convert them into safer estriol.

"Estrogen balance is impossible to maintain when there is iodine deficiency present," writes Dr. Brownstein.

Breast cancer

Now that we've established the incontrovertible link between iodine and estrogen balance, it's easy to see how a lack of sufficient iodine and bromine interference causes runaway estrogen levels leading to breast cancer.

Bernard Eskin, M.D., of Drexel University in Philadelphia, one of the foremost researchers in the field of iodine and breast cancer, conducted animal research in the field for more than 40 years. His work gives us some pivotal basic truths about iodine and breast health:

1. Long-term iodine depletion causes changes in breast tissue.

2. When sufficient iodine is added to the diet, breast tissue returns to its normal state.

3. Normal iodine intake results in normal estrogen function in breast tissue.

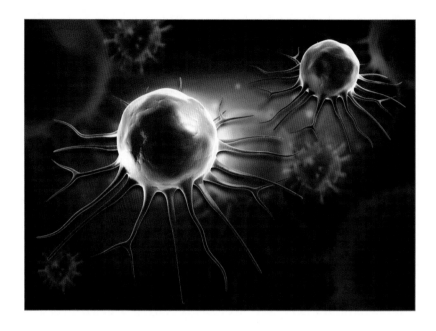

4. Iodine supplementation blocked the development of cancer in animals given cancer-causing substances.

5. Molecular iodine, like that found in kelp and other forms of seaweed, is the most effective form of the mineral for the treatment of all types of breast disease. However, most people do not have kelp in their normal diets, and the amount in kelp varies according to conditions. In addition, laboratory testing has shown high concentrations of heavy metals in kelp and other sea vegetables. That is why it is better to use a supplement when dealing with specific diseases that respond to iodine.

Here are more exciting research results showing the connection between low iodine levels in the body and breast cancer:

1. Iodine supplementation desensitized estrogen receptors in breast tissue, meaning iodine gets to cells where it is needed rather than being "bumped" by toxic bromines.

2. Iodine caused cancer cell death (apoptosis is the medical term) rather than wild reproduction of cells characteristic of cancers of all types.

3. It also caused more cancer cell death than the commonly used chemotherapy drug, Fluorouracil, also known as 5-FU, which has numerous and debilitating side effects.

Iodine has also been shown to increase the activity of the BRCA1 gene that helps balance estrogen activity in breast tissues and even to increase the effectiveness of the breast cancer drug tamoxifen and decrease resistance to tamoxifen.

Throughout this book, I've mentioned several types of iodine: potassium iodide, sodium iodide and molecular iodine from kelp. A great deal of research suggests that molecular iodine is particularly helpful in established estrogen balance and even reversing breast cancer.

Several studies show that adding seaweed to rats' diets reduced the rate of breast tumors, stopped the growth of existing tumors and caused cell death in three known breast cancer cell lines, leading Dr. Brownstein to write, "You cannot give breast cancer to rats that have sufficient iodine."

Whenever I do a lecture on iodine, I am asked about dosages and whether 12.5 mg or more isn't too much. Years ago, we thought that 400 IU of vitamin D a day was more than adequate. Yet we live in a toxic world that is more toxic today than it was just 20 years ago.

Iodine is going along the same path as vitamin D. There is no research showing that 150 mcg of iodine is sufficient and our exposure to Black Hat halogens is far more than ever before in history. We live in a chemical environment and we need more vitamins and minerals.

Bear in mind that dosage levels vary. Your thyroid alone needs approximately 5 mg of iodine per day, but since we know that iodine is used by the cells of the breast, ovaries, uterus and prostate, higher dosages are warranted for almost everyone. A useful dosage for an adult would be 12.5 mg—that's enough to keep your thyroid functioning and to help the other iodine-hungry tissues, including breast, ovaries and skin. For the higher dosage of iodine, recommended by holistic physicians, you're looking at up to 50 mg per day based on an iodine loading test. The higher doses are often done under the supervision of integrative practitioners. (See Chapter 8.)

Dr. Guy Abraham, a UCLA professor, pioneer in iodine therapy and leader of the Iodine Project that researched the many needs for and uses of iodine in the human body, was a proponent of iodine supplementation to prevent breast cancer. He said it takes 20 to 40 times the amount of iodine to control fibrocystic disease and breast cancer than it does to control goiter.

For people with breast cancer, daily dosages as high as 100 mg of iodine are often appropriate. Don't do this without medical supervision. Discuss iodine supplementation with your doctor and monitor it regularly.

Dr. Abraham noted that iodine supplements have been taken for breast cancer in quantities as high as 6 *grams* a day without negative effects.

CHAPTER 5

Iodine and Other Forms of Cancer

et's make this chapter short and simple: Everything I've said about iodine and breast cancer applies to any hormonally related cancer, including ovarian, uterine, endometrial, prostate, thyroid and pancreatic.

The same rules especially apply to all cancers that are related to excess estrogen: breast, endometrial, ovarian and uterine.

Iodine protects against a variety of types of cancers, but when iodine can't get into the cells, you are vulnerable.

Iodine is not absorbed by the cells and is unable to protect them primarily because iodine absorption is blocked by the toxic halogens: chlorine, fluorine and bromine, all of them proven to trigger various types of cancer. We know that toxic halogens, those Black Hat halogens, are everywhere in our diet and in our environment. We find bromine in anything made with flour, and we find chlorine in all municipal drinking water. Fluorine or fluoride is found in many sources of municipal drinking water and toothpastes and mouthwashes. It's very difficult, perhaps impossible, to avoid them.

There's another problem with bromine. The International Agency for Research on Cancer classified potassium bromate as a

Group 2B carcinogen, and it was banned in the U.K. in 1990 and in Canada in 1994. Sadly, it's still legal in the U.S., although in 1999 the Center for Science in the Public Interest (CSPI) petitioned the FDA to ban it, saying the agency "has known for years that bromate causes cancer in laboratory animals."

Now add in the modern-day scourge of cancer-causing environmental estrogens, also called xenoestrogens. They're found in:

- Plastics, many of which contain phthalates and bisphenol A, proven carcinogens

- Pesticides and weed killers with glyphosates (RoundUp™), DDT, atrazine and a host of other chemicals

- Meat and dairy products that contain hormone-disrupting growth hormones

- Soy that contains natural estrogenic compounds

- Personal-care products like shampoos, cosmetics and laundry detergents that contain phthalates, lauryl sulfate, BHA and BHT, DEA, parabens, PEG compounds, petrolatum and many more

- Sunscreens and other skin-care products with parabens

- Birth control pills that contain ethinyl estradiol

- Children's sleepwear with fire-retardant polybrominated diphenyl ethers (PBDEs)

- Cookware made with Teflon

- Anything made with propyl gallate, which may include all sorts of food products, hair products, even chewing gum, adhesives and lubricants

- Shrimp and shellfish preserved with the preservative 4-hexylresorcinol, which is often not labeled

There are many, many more. But I think you get the idea. I had a friend who decided she would avoid all plastics for a year. She pledged not to buy anything packaged in plastic or use any plastic containers for an entire year. An entire year! Ha! She gave up in utter frustration after just two weeks. Her organic meat was wrapped in plastic-coated paper at the health food store, the organic veggies were encased in plastic cocoons and the organic shampoo was sold in—you guessed it—a plastic bottle. And that was just the intention to avoid the environmental estrogens in plastic!

As you can see from the list above, it is quite literally impossible to avoid xenoestrogens. They are in our food, our water, our furniture, our clothing, the air we breathe and the water we drink.

Dr. Brownstein writes, after examining the omnipresence of estrogenic toxins in our environment, "It is no wonder that hormone-sensitive cancers like breast (as well as prostate and uterine) cancer have reached epidemic proportions."

But he adds that the positive effects of iodine in converting malignant breast tissue into normal tissue is true for all other hormonally related cancers.

Early research by Dr. Guy Abraham confirms that iodine may protect against cancer of the breast, ovaries, prostate, uterus and thyroid gland. I would add pancreatic cancer to that list. Dr. Abraham believes that iodine works as an antioxidant, reducing damage to DNA, and that it affects the pituitary, hypothalamus, thyroid and adrenal glands, all of which regulate hormones.

Ovaries contain the second highest iodine levels, after the thyroid. Russian studies done several years ago showed a relationship between iodine deficiency and the presence of cysts in the ovaries. The greater the iodine deficiency, the more ovarian cysts a woman produces. In its extreme form, this condition is known as polycystic ovary syndrome (PCOS), which increases the risk of ovarian cancer.

Thyroid cancer

Thyroid cancer is another matter. It doesn't seem to be directly related to estrogen, but Dr. Jorge D. Flechas, an internationally respected iodine proponent who practices family medicine in Hendersonville, NC, notes, "In those areas of the world where iodine deficiency is very problematic, such as in Switzerland and in certain areas of Asia and Africa, there are also higher incidences of thyroid cancer."

I'll add French Polynesia to that list as well as a wide variety of locations where residents are known to have low iodine intake, such as the so-called Goiter Belt around the Great Lakes region of the United States, where the soil is low in iodine.

People who have goiters are more likely to get thyroid cancer than those who do not. By now, you have no doubt figured out that low iodine levels are once again the link.

Thyroid cancer rates have tripled since 1975, according to shocking new research from the Veterans Administration in collaboration

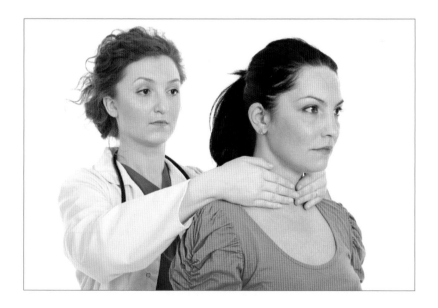

with Dartmouth Institute for Health Policy. That is a 300% increase! Researchers termed these thyroid cancer statistics an "epidemic."

> It takes 20 to 40 times the amount of iodine
> needed to control breast cancer and fibrocystic
> disease than it does to prevent goiter.

As Dr. Flechas tells us, lumps, bumps, cysts and nodules seem to be routine in people with low iodine levels, and they are common symptoms in a variety of conditions that can lead to cancer, including fibrocystic breasts, thyroid nodules and goiters.

A study published in the *Journal of the American College of Surgeons* sheds some interesting light on the subject, confirming that people with thyroid nodules have an 18% higher risk of thyroid cancer. But a side finding was even more interesting: People with Graves' disease, one of the forms of hyperthyroidism, which is not linked to low iodine, had no greater risk of thyroid cancer.

That says to me, and it should say to you, that low iodine is undoubtedly linked to thyroid cancer and several other types of cancer. That is sufficient reason for me to take a close look at iodine levels and to ensure that those levels are optimal to prevent all of these problems, especially in the presence of bromine.

Can supplemental iodine cause thyroid cancer? The answer is an unequivocal, "No!"

Radioactive iodine, the most commonly used "therapy" for hyperthyroidism (overactive thyroid) can and does cause thyroid cancer. The remedy for radioactive iodine poisoning? Potassium iodide—the good iodine used universally to neutralize the radioactive version. More about that in Chapter 7.

Other types of cancer

Let's step back and talk about goiters again. In 1924, 90 years ago, researchers found that people who had goiters were far more likely to develop gastrointestinal cancer, including stomach and eso-phageal cancers. In fact, that same pivotal study found that European countries with the highest rates of goiter also had the highest death rates from all types of cancers.

In 2000, Italian researchers theorized that iodine functions as an antioxidant in the stomach lining, which protects against cancer.

A 2012 study from the George Washington University Cancer Institute in Washington, D.C., took the theory a step farther. It's a little complicated, so bear with me. In the embryonic stage, the thyroid gland and the stomach have similar origins in the foregut. Both organs concentrate iodine. Researchers found that chronic inflammation and the tissue destruction that accompanies inflammation (often from environmental sources) in one organ (like the thyroid) can trigger cancer in a distant organ (like the stomach or esophagus that are developmentally related tissues).

While science still doesn't tell us why, it does tell us how low iodine levels can cause gastrointestinal cancers: The low iodine levels in the thyroid somehow signal the linings of the stomach and esophagus (gastric mucosa), creating gastritis, a painful but benign condition that has a tendency to become cancerous. What's even more enlightening is that the researchers theorize that the same may hold true for the link between iodine deficiency and many other types of cancer.

Low iodine levels also cause achlorhydria (lack of digestive acid production). Iodine is used by the stomach cells to concentrate chloride, which is necessary to produce hydrochloric acid (digestive acid). Long-term impairment of stomach acid production dramatically escalates the risk of stomach cancer.

Beyond the gastric cancers, iodine plays a very strong role in the production of lymph and the health of the entire lymphatic system that sweeps toxins out of the body. When your lymphatic system is working properly, it eliminates large quantities of all types of toxins, including those that can cause cancer. It takes optimal iodine levels for the lymphatic system to do its job.

Other Benefits

The Weston A. Price Foundation theorizes that iodine may be helpful in treating other types of cancer because it triggers apoptosis, programmed cell death. All normal cells have a normal lifespan. They are born and they die. For unknown reasons, cancer cells become immortal or near-immortal. They reproduce wildly and don't die, so tumors grow and eventually obstruct vital organs. Any substance that causes these cells to return to their normal lifespan and die on cue is going to help fight cancer.

In one important study, human lung cancer cells with genes spliced into them that enhance iodine uptake converted to apoptosis and shrank when given iodine, both when grown in labs and implanted in mice.

Some other body tissues actually concentrate iodine through a natural process called the iodine pump. This pump is more like a concentrator that works in combination with sodium (another of many reasons not to restrict sodium intake). We know that iodine plays an important role in these organs—the stomach mucosa, salivary glands, ovaries, thymus gland, skin, brain, joints, arteries and bone—and it stands to reason that the iodine pump can help protect these organs from cancer or stop uncontrolled cell division if cancer occurs.

Many practitioners are now advocating wider use for iodine in treating and preventing cancer.

CHAPTER 6

Iodine and Children

*I*odine deficiency is the leading cause of preventable mental retardation worldwide.

I'm repeating this sobering fact first mentioned in Chapter 1
because it is so horrifying. What if a pregnant woman consumed a
handful of pills that costs a few cents and protected her baby
against mental deficiency and a crippling disease called cretinism?
That's all it takes to prevent this tragedy of epic proportions.

Iodine deficiency affects pregnant women, their babies and
children in alarming numbers.

Let's start at the beginning.

Women of childbearing age

Women with severe iodine deficiency are at risk for infertility, and,
if they do become pregnant, they are at a higher risk for miscar-
riage, stillbirth, preterm delivery and birth defects in their babies,
according to the National Institutes of Health (NIH).

Pregnancy depletes the mother's mineral stores, including
iodine, which is why pregnant women need at least 50% more
iodine to help give the baby the minerals it needs.

Newly released research from the National Health and Nutrition Examination Survey (NHANES) confirms that women of

reproductive age have the lowest iodine levels of all adults, barely above the markers for iodine deficiency. The American Academy of Pediatrics recently released a new policy statement urging the use of supplemental iodine for pregnant and breastfeeding women, pointing out that currently only 15% of women are taking supplements that contain adequate levels of iodine.

It's disturbing to note that not all prenatal vitamins widely used in the United States contain iodine, even though the American Thyroid Association recommends minimal iodine dosages—150 mcg daily—for all pregnant women and nursing mothers. The Institute of Medicine recommends 220 mcg a day for pregnant women and 290 mcg daily for nursing mothers. Even the staid National Institutes of Health (NIH) says that up to 1,100 mcg of iodine is "likely safe" for pregnant and lactating women.

The Linus Pauling Institute warns that iodine deficiency during pregnancy can be a serious health problem for the mother, leading to potentially life-threatening preeclampsia, high blood pressure during pregnancy.

For fetuses, newborns and infants

Sufficient iodine is essential for brain development in fetuses and young children. Hypothyroidism in children has serious permanent effects on the brain if it is untreated, and even mild cases can detract from cognitive development.

The World Health Organization estimates that there are 285 million school-age children worldwide who are iodine deficient.

Breastfed infants get iodine from breast milk. However, the iodine content of breast milk depends on how much iodine the mother gets.

The effects of even mild iodine deficiency during pregnancy and in the early years of a child's life can have profoundly negative effects on brain development and can doom a child to a lifetime of diminished intelligence.

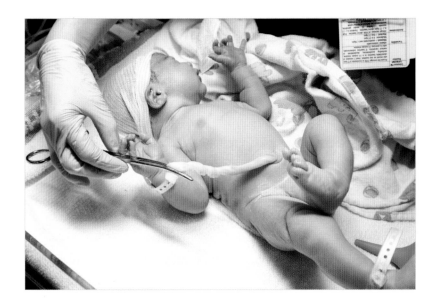

Iodine plays a crucial role in the development of the brain and other parts of the central nervous system. Iodine deficiency during pregnancy can lead to a condition called congenital hypothyroidism, or low thyroid function from before birth. Congenital hypothyroidism can permanently compromise the child's mental development and, in severe cases, leads to mental retardation, dwarfism and cretinism.

Cretinism is caused by severe iodine deficiency during pregnancy. Children with cretinism suffer from permanent brain damage, mental retardation, deaf mutism, spasticity and short stature. Fortunately, this sort of severe iodine deficiency and its tragic results is rarely seen in the Western world, but it is common in areas of Asia and Africa with low soil iodine levels.

Sadly, iodine supplementation after a baby is born with mental impairment or cretinism will not reverse the problem, says the NIH.

Even without congenital hypothyroidism, iodine deficiency during infancy may result in abnormal brain development and impaired intellectual development, says the Linus Pauling Institute.

Even a mild iodine deficiency during pregnancy, like that which affects about half of our population, has been shown to result in children with IQs that are more than 10 points lower than their counterparts born of iodine sufficient mothers.

One study showed that children born in iodine-deficient areas had IQs that were 11 points lower than those born in iodine-sufficient areas. As Dr. Brownstein notes, "An 11-point decline in IQ can mean the difference between a successful child and a troubled child."

The NIH adds that although children of mothers from iodine-deficient regions may have normal thyroid function test results, they have been documented with lower language and memory performance.

Iodine deficiency in children and adolescents is often associated with goiter. The incidence of goiter peaks in adolescence and is more common in girls. School children in iodine-deficient areas show poorer school performance, lower IQs and a higher incidence of learning disabilities than matched groups from iodine-sufficient areas. One review of 18 studies concluded that iodine deficiency alone lowered mean IQ scores in children by 13.5 points.

Several recent studies link autism in children to iodine deficiency in their mothers. One from Weill Cornell Medical College in New York shows a fourfold increase in the risk of autism in children of mothers with severe iodine deficiency.

Given the fact that about 1% of the world's population suffers from some impairment on the autism spectrum, researchers would be well advised to take a further look at the role iodine deficiency and bromine toxicity might be playing in the escalating number of children with autism.

The National Institutes of Health adds that mental retardation as a result of iodine deficiency can be made worse if the mother is deficient in selenium, a trace mineral crucial in brain and thyroid development. Vitamin D is also crucial to brain development and shortfalls may worsen the effects of iodine. Vitamin D shortfalls have also been linked to the rising autism rates.

Environmental factors

Iodine deficiency in the mother increases sensitivity to certain environmental toxins, particularly thiocyanates, iodine-blocking chemicals found in cruciferous vegetables like broccoli and tobacco smoke that act much like toxic halogens. Some research suggests that low iodine levels also increase sensitivity to perchlorate, a toxic chemical used in rocket fuel, fireworks and flares that is found in 4% of all public drinking water supplies.

Reversible iodine deficiency problems in children

Iodine deficiency in infants through the elementary school years can lead to behavioral problems, poor school performance and, according to Dr. Brownstein, can set the stage for lifelong learning problems.

ADHD

ADHD (attention deficit and hyperactivity disorder) is another epidemic in today's world. The Centers for Disease Control and Prevention (CDC) says ADHD is the most common neurobehavioral disorder of children, with its numbers steadily escalating to

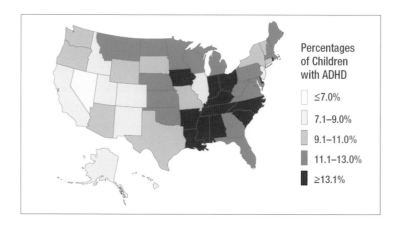

as high as 18.7% in children between the ages of 8 and 17. These latest figures end in 2011, but given the unrelenting increase in ADHD diagnoses in the past 11 years, it wouldn't be out of place to assume the numbers continue to escalate.

It's also interesting to note that some of the states with the highest numbers of children with ADHD are the former Goiter Belt around the Great Lakes, where historically soils have been low in iodine.

Dr. Brownstein says that every child with a diagnosis of ADD/ADHD should have a complete nutritional and hormonal evaluation. He is convinced that many, if not most, of these children are actually suffering from iodine deficiency, which is easily corrected.

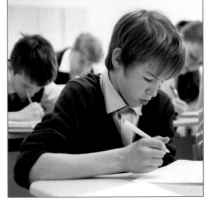

ADHD is not caused by a deficiency of Ritalin or other prescription drugs given to children to suppress the symptoms of the disorder, says Dr. Brownstein.

"ADHD is caused by nutrient and hormonal imbalances, including iodine deficiency," he asserts.

Closely monitored iodine supplementation in children with ADHD has been shown to reverse the effects, resolve behavioral problems and improve learning abilities.

Infants and young children are very sensitive to fluctuations in their iodine levels. Low levels of iodine put them at risk for poor mental and psychomotor development, especially in language and memory skills. Some of these children may even be diagnosed with mental retardation.

The good news is that for these children, who were not deprived of iodine in utero, iodine supplementation and thyroid hormone replacement have been known to reverse the problem.

Toxic halogens

The worldwide epidemic of iodine deficiency applies to children as well and increases their need for more iodine in view of the pervasive toxic halogens—bromine, chlorine and fluorine—everywhere in our environment.

Research has linked iodine supplementation with increased ability of iodine to use the iodine receptors and knock the Black Hat halogens off their perches so life-giving iodine can be utilized.

WHO'S RECOMMENDED IODINE INTAKE	
Preschool children (0–59 months)	90 mcg
School-age children (6–12 years)	120 mcg
Adults (above 12 years)	150 mcg
Pregnant and lactating women	200 mcg

Testing and supplements for children

Children can be tested for iodine sufficiency with a 24-hour urine test in the same way adults are tested, but at a lower dosage depending on their weight.

Supplemental iodine can be very helpful for children, but you must work with a qualified medical practitioner who can do the appropriate testing and monitoring.

Dr. Brownstein thinks these requirements are far too low and recommends iodine intake based on weight at 0.11 mg per pound per day, so a 50-pound child should get 5.5 mg (milligrams) of iodine daily.

CHAPTER 7

Iodine, Detoxification and Other Health Conditions

This is a bit of a catch-all chapter. I'm going to give you the formula to help detoxify your body of those Black Hat halogens and mention a few of the other health challenges that are related to low iodine levels.

Detoxification

If you've read this far, you already understand that iodine shortfalls are closely linked to those toxic Black Hat halogens that rob your body of its ability to absorb the iodine it so desperately needs.

You also know that most of us are exposed to these toxins every day of our lives. It is difficult to avoid them.

So we all want to know how to detoxify ourselves of those Black Hat halogens and improve our ability to absorb iodine.

Here's a simple checklist:

❏ Take a good quality iodine supplement, preferably one that contains potassium iodide, sodium iodide and a molecular form of iodine from sea vegetables. The high doses of iodine will help your body release the toxic halogens. Your health practitioner should be able to help you determine dosage. Most people need 12.5 mg up to 50 mg, but people with cancer may need even more.

❏ Use unrefined sea salt to help rid your body of bromine and rebalance your overall mineral status. Dr. Brownstein recommends 1 to 1.5 teaspoons daily. You can help the detoxification process by adding $1/4$ to $1/2$ tsp of Celtic sea salt with one quart of water and drinking three quarts of this mixture daily to help draw out the toxic halogens.

❏ Drink lots of water to help flush out the toxins. Drink clean filtered water that is free of chlorine or fluoride. A whole house water filter or an under-the-sink filter will do the job nicely. Cold-pressed charcoal filters are the best. There are also hand-held versions of water purifiers, some used for camping or emergency needs. The best are those used by the military. I'm not really in favor of reverse osmosis water filters because they remove nearly all minerals from the water. The easy water intake calculation: Divide your body weight by 2: So if you weigh 150 pounds, you need 75 ounces of water a day. You need more in hot weather and when you're exercising heavily.

❏ Take vitamin C, a powerful antioxidant that stimulates detoxification. Use only whole food molecular vitamin C, the most effective because it contains all of the dozens of components of vitamin C, not just ascorbic acid. Start with 1,000 mg and go up as high as 3,000 mg daily.

Detoxification can be slightly unpleasant, but don't give up. In rare cases, some people experience pimples, skin rashes or redness. These are signs that the toxic halogens are being released from your body. If you feel tired or achy, that means the detoxification is working. Drink more water, take more whole food vitamin C and most importantly, don't give up! The detox blues will pass, I promise!

Diabetes

Correct iodine levels have been studied and proven to improve

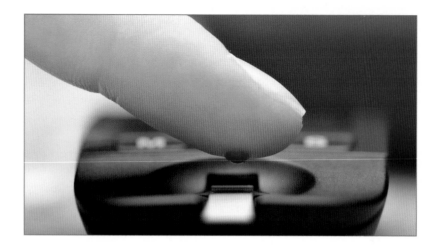

blood glucose control in people diagnosed with type 2 diabetes. Furthermore, correct iodine levels can also minimize the risk of the heart disease that often goes hand in hand with diabetes.

"Iodine attaches to insulin receptors and improves glucose metabolism, which is good news for people with diabetes," says iodine researcher Michael Donaldson, Ph.D., of Hallelujah Acres Lifestyle Centers.

Heart disease

Diabetes and heart disease are closely linked. Since we know that diabetes is linked to low iodine, we can also forge the connection between low iodine levels and heart disease.

Recent research from the University of British Columbia confirms the link between iodine insufficiency and cardiovascular disease.

Dr. Donaldson says, "Iodine stabilizes the heart rhythm, lowers serum cholesterol, lowers blood pressure, and is known to make the blood thinner. Iodine is not only good for the cardiovascular system, it is vital. Sufficient iodine is needed for a stable rhythmic heart beat."

Joint and muscle pain

Joint and muscle pain, chronic fatigue and fibromyalgia have all been linked to hypothyroidism. By extrapolation, they are closely linked to iodine shortfalls.

Muscle pain and achiness have been reported in medical literature for more than 100 years, and doctors have reported improvement in the symptoms of fibromyalgia when thyroid deficiency is treated.

People with chronic fatigue and immune dysfunction syndrome (CFIDS) and fibromyalgia often share a basket of symptoms that almost always include muscle pain, joint pain and profound fatigue. In his book *Overcoming Thyroid Disorders*, Dr. David Brownstein notes that numerous studies show that many people with fibromyalgia and CFIDS also have hypothyroidism.

One study put that number at 63% and another at 50%, and Dr. Brownstein writes that his experiences with patients with fibromyalgia and CFIDS shows that more than 80% have clinically validated hypothyroidism.

Conventional medicine doesn't recognize this link, says Dr. Brownstein, because doctors rely on the TSH (thyroid-stimulating hormone) test alone to diagnose the disease. That test is woefully insufficient, so relatively few people are actually correctly diagnosed with hypothyroidism.

"It is my belief that, in many individuals, fibromyalgia develops as a chronic disorder after a long period of untreated hypothyroidism," Dr. Brownstein writes.

Other thyroid experts have noted that the rise in diagnoses of CFIDS and fibromyalgia coincide with the time the TSH test came into widespread use in 1980, leaving large numbers of patients with undiagnosed hypothyroidism.

Fortunately, fibromyalgia can often be reversed when thyroid insufficiency is treated—and it's most often treated with iodine and thyroid hormones.

Antimicrobial

Grandma used it on every cut and sore, quite effectively, but also quite painfully.

Iodine is still used today in hospitals to prevent infection, particularly before surgery, when surgical sites are liberally painted with an iodine solution.

Supplemental iodine has strong antimicrobial effects without the sting.

Dr. Guy Abraham says, "In sufficient amounts, iodine can not only adjust a dysfunctional thyroid, it can assist with a host of glandular imbalances as well as a wide assortment of internal as well as external bacteria, fungi and viruses. Iodine has many non-endocrine biologic effects, including the role it plays in the physiology of the inflammatory response. Iodides increase the movement of granulocytes into areas of inflammation and improve the phagocytosis of bacteria by granulocytes and the ability of granulocytes to kill bacteria."

That's just fancy medical lingo for, "It works!"

Asthma and lung disease

Several studies show that supplemental amounts of iodine can reduce viscous bronchial secretions in adults and children with asthma. The research suggests that iodine helps calm the autoimmune response that triggers asthma attacks

"By keeping the mucous membranes healthy, iodine greatly helps to overcome autoimmune diseases, sinus problems, asthma, lung cancer, and other lung problems, and also intestinal diseases, including inflammatory conditions, and cancers," writes Walter Last, author of *The Natural Way to Heal.*

Alzheimer's and Parkinson's diseases

Researchers from the University of Victoria, British Columbia, created a fascinating theory of the "disease family tree," hypothesizing that deficiencies of iodine lead to what appears to be hereditary disease in families.

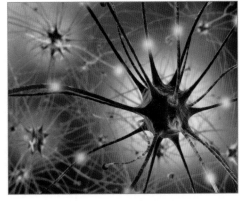

They wrote in a pivotal 1987 study, "Deficiencies of this essential trace element appear to be associated with many diseases, or birth defects, including goiter, cretinism, multiple sclerosis, amyotrophic lateral sclerosis and cancer of the thyroid and nervous system."

They continued, "Although the evidence is weaker, iodine deficiency may also be implicated in Alzheimer's and Parkinson's diseases."

Insufficient iodine appears to interfere with the body's ability to manufacture brain chemicals. Later research shows that Parkinson's and ALS, both diseases affecting the dopamine receptors in the brain, occur more frequently in low-iodine areas. A study published in the *Journal of Orthomolecular Medicine* in 1999 suggests that long-term iodine deficiency permanently impairs the dopamine receptors in the brain, opening a pathway for neurological diseases.

Inability to sweat and risk of heatstroke

Since 20% of the body's iodine stores are located in the skin, low iodine levels impair the body's ability to sweat. When you can't sweat, you get overheated and risk a heatstroke, which can be life threatening.

Radiation detoxification

Worries about radiation poisoning are not far from the forefront of our consciousness these days since the tsunami in Japan destroyed a nuclear power plant, releasing untold amounts of radiation.

Potassium iodide (the iconic KI) is the go-to remedy to protect thyroids against radiation exposure in conventional medicine and in integrative medicine today, and for good reason: It works.

Here's how: When sufficient healthy iodine is used, the thyroid and other receptors become saturated, leaving no room for radioactive iodine to take hold.

I know that people who live near nuclear power plants in Southern California have been given potassium iodide tablets to keep in their homes and to be used when directed if there is a nuclear accident. I hope that is enough and that it's all they need.

As I mentioned before, potassium iodide is also used to stop the toxic effects of radioactive iodine used to "kill" thyroids of people who have extreme forms of hyperthyroidism (overactive thyroid). If your iodine levels are correct, radioactive iodine will have minimal effect.

Migraines

Many migraine headaches are triggered by hormonal fluctuations. While most often these are sex hormone swings, particularly in women, any hormone, including thyroid hormone, can play a role in causing migraines. Of course, we already know that low iodine intake causes hypothyroidism or low thyroid function, so it's not at all a leap of logic to look at insufficient iodine as a trigger for migraines. Preliminary evidence indicates that there may be a connection between thyroid abnormalities and migraine headaches, but more research is needed to better understand this connection.

CHAPTER 8

The Right Iodine

Are you iodine deficient?

If you've experienced the symptoms mentioned in the questionnaire on page 7, you may be iodine deficient. Of course, many of these symptoms could apply to many health challenges. Fatigue, weight gain, digestive complaints, fibrocystic breast disease and more can have multiple causes.

I'll go out on a limb and say this: You are almost certainly iodine deficient and/or bromine toxic if you've been diagnosed with hypothyroidism or, since conventional medicine is lamentably poor at diagnosing this common condition, even if you suspect you have it.

Iodine testing

Hypothyroidism alone is a reason to test for iodine deficiency.

If your self-test shows you need more iodine, you'll need to do the 24-hour iodine loading urine test.

Drs. Flechas, Brownstein and Abraham firmly believe that this test is the only definitive test of iodine levels.

You'll take 50 mg of iodine and carefully collect all urine for 24 hours, according to your doctor's instructions.

The principle behind the iodine loading test, according to Dr. Brownstein, is that if the body has sufficient iodine, one would expect that all or most of the 50 mg of iodine you've taken in would be excreted in the urine. If not, then more of the iodine would be retained.

If you are iodine sufficient, 45 mg or more of that iodine load will be excreted in your urine. If you excrete less than 90% of the iodine, supplements can bring you up to par.

DIY IODINE TESTING

You can get an idea of your levels with an easy at-home test. All you need is a bottle of tincture of iodine (sold in pharmacies) and a cotton ball.

Here's how:

1. On your clean forearm, swab a circle of the bronzy-orange iodine solution, roughly 2 inches in diameter.

2. Leave it undisturbed for 24 hours.

Results, according to Dr. Abraham:

- If the stain disappears in less than eight hours, you desperately need iodine.

- If it disappears in 24 hours, you also need iodine.

- If it simply stays on your arm and begins to slowly fade in color after a full 24 hours, you have already reached iodine sufficiency.

Please note that while this test is quite useful, age and certain skin conditions as well as atmospheric pressure may interfere with the results. Therefore, if you try the cotton ball/iodine test and it shows you are sufficient, yet you still have symptoms, you may need to see an integrative practitioner for deeper evaluation and/or to perform the iodine loading test.

Iodine in your diet

Most of us don't get anywhere near enough iodine in our diets. Iodized salt, as I mentioned in Chapter 1, does little or nothing to improve our levels. For decades, we've known that our soils cannot give us enough of this essential mineral through crops grown in iodine-depleted soils.

The Japanese, with a food culture rich in seafood and sea vegetables, probably have the highest iodine levels of any population. The Japanese government reports an average intake of 13.8 mg of iodine daily through diet alone, but noted that Japanese people who live in non-coastal areas have significantly lower iodine intake at an average of 5.3 mg daily.

On Japan's island of Okinawa, there are more people over the age of 100 than anywhere else on Earth. It has been reported that their diets include 80 to 200 mg of iodine daily.

Without eating substantial amounts of seaweed, it is nearly impossible to get more than 1 mg of iodine through diet alone.

For most Americans, food intake of iodine is simply not enough to produce optimal levels of iodine—or optimal health. Neither is it enough to protect us from the toxic Black Hat halogens!

Iodine supplements

Iodine you consume in foods and supplements is excreted from the body in 24 to 48 hours, which means daily consumption or supplementation of iodine is critical for health.

For most of us, this means an iodine supplement is the sole means of maintaining optimal iodine levels.

So which supplement is the best choice?

I have chosen a triple iodine/iodide formulation that I believe provides the most absorbable forms of iodine. It contains potassium iodide, sodium iodide and molecular iodine from kelp. Let's take a brief look at each one and its importance.

Potassium and sodium iodide

Potassium and sodium iodide are the forms of iodine best used by the thyroid.

Molecular iodine (from kelp)

A review paper examining results obtained in studies of breast health noted that while all forms tested (molecular iodine, sodium iodide and potassium iodide) produced beneficial effects, the best results for breast support were achieved with molecular iodine.

How much?

This is the $64,000 question! Your iodine loading test will tell you what your levels are.

Dosage levels vary, depending on the magnitude of your shortfall (assuming almost everyone has a shortfall!). Your thyroid alone needs approximately 5 mg of iodine per day, but since we know that iodine is used by the cells of the breast, ovaries, uterus, prostate and pancreas, higher dosages are warranted for almost everyone.

A maintenance dosage for an adult would be 12.5 mg. For the higher dosage of iodine, recommended by holistic physicians, you're looking at up to 50 mg per day. For people with breast cancer, possibly 100 mg of iodine per day is appropriate, although I would urge you to discuss this with your integrative practitioner. Dr. Brownstein tells me he takes 75 mg per day. I take 50 mg per day.

Before the advent of the synthetic drugs that are used today, iodine was one of the most beneficial and universal medicines used by physicians around the world. It was effective for everything: healing wounds and disease, destroying bacteria, viruses and pathogens and even preventing cancer. But iodine was soon forgotten in favor of new pharmaceutical drugs. Now we're seeing the

FOOD SOURCES OF IODINE

Food	Micrograms (mcg) per serving	Percent DV*
Seaweed, whole or sheet, 1 g	16–2,984	11%–1,989%
Cod, baked, 3 ounces	99	66%
Milk, whole, 1 cup	81	55%
Yogurt, plain, low-fat, 1 cup	75	50%
Iodized salt, 1.5 g (approx. $1/4$ tsp)	71	47%
Shrimp, 3 ounces	35	23%
Ice cream, chocolate, $1/2$ cup	30	20%
Macaroni, enriched, boiled, 1 cup	27	18%
Egg, 1 large	24	16%
Tuna, canned in oil, drained, 3 ounces	17	11%
Prunes, dried, 5 prunes	13	9%
Cheese, cheddar, 1 ounce	12	8%
Raisin bran cereal, 1 cup	11	7%
Lima beans, mature, boiled, $1/2$ cup	8	5%
Apple juice, 1 cup	7	5%
Green peas, frozen, boiled, $1/2$ cup	3	2%
Banana, 1 medium	3	2%

Source: National Institutes of Health Office of Dietary Supplements

*DV = Daily Value. DVs were developed by the U.S. Food and Drug Administration (FDA) to help consumers compare the nutrient contents of products within the context of a total diet. The DV for iodine is 150 mcg for adults and children aged 4 and older. However, the FDA does not require food labels to list iodine content unless a food has been fortified with this nutrient. Foods providing 20% or more of the DV are considered to be high sources of a nutrient.

Author's note: The USDA's Daily Values are simply the levels needed to prevent goiter. This level does not come close to providing for the needs of the rest of the body or begin to counteract the levels of toxic halogens.

painful result—skyrocketing cancer rates, an epidemic of thyroid dysfunction, neuropsychiatric disorders and serious problems detoxifying our bodies.

Drs. Abraham and Brownstein believe that because of widespread bromide and fluoride toxicity, many people today actually need up to 50 mg of iodine daily, amounts we can get with supplements. I agree wholeheartedly. But, almost anyone would benefit from a daily dose of 6.25 mg or 12.5 mg.

Too much?

Of course, these levels are substantially higher than the DV recommend by the government and even far above the Institute of Medicine's Tolerable Upper Intake Levels of about 1,100 mcg for adults.

Dr. Gabriel Cousens of the Tree of Life Rejuvenation Center in Patagonia, AZ, an M.D., homeopath and pioneer in the holistic health movement in the United States says, "Historically, as early as 1911, people normally took between 300–900 mg daily without incident. How is it that now only 1/5,000th of this dose is now considered safe? Even the Food and Nutritional Board at the Institute of Medicine has set the tolerable upper limit of 1,100 micrograms of iodine daily. Other researchers have used between 300 and 600 mg/day to prevent goiter. Iodine is found in every single one of our body's hundred trillion cells. Without adequate iodine levels life is impossible. Iodine is the universal health nutrient and brings health on many levels."

So is it safe to take iodine at these levels? You'll find as many opinions on the subject as there are "experts," but I trust Guy Abraham and David Brownstein, the doctors I know who have looked into the subject more deeply than anyone else on the planet.

They have treated thousands of patients with doses of iodine hundreds, even thousands, of times greater than the government's daily values or tolerable upper limits, all without serious side effects.

ADDITIONAL SUPPLEMENTS
TO ENHANCE ABSORPTION OF IODINE

Since enhanced iodine absorption is a key factor here, there is an excellent blend of nutrients that will do just that. I highly recommend that you add the following formula to your iodine supplement.

Selenium: 200 mcg

This trace mineral found in the soil has sometimes been called the missing link in treating hypothyroidism. Selenium acts synergistically with iodine, meaning each enhances the effectiveness of the other in promoting iodine's availability to the cells. Selenium also protects the thyroid from oxidative stress that can occur when iodide is converted to iodine. It is a component of the enzyme that helps convert T4 to T3. Some experts say low T3 levels are common in areas with selenium-poor soils and crops.

When there is an iodine deficiency, supplementing with selenium will magnify the iodine deficiency causing it to become worse. In fact, any time either selenium or iodine levels are high and the other is low, symptoms will occur and oftentimes worsen. If there is a deficiency, both must be supplemented and brought into balance. Selenium deficiency can aggravate Hashimoto's hypothyroidism (an autoimmune disease) as well as other thyroid disorders. Selenium supplementation has also been shown to reduce the thyroid antibodies associated with this disorder. Selenium-rich foods include kidney, liver, beef, chicken, turkey, crab, other shellfish, eggs, mushrooms, onions, brown rice, barley, oats, Brazil nuts and sunflower seeds.

Thiamine: 100 mg

Also known as B1, thiamine is critical for many of the steps leading to the synthesis and activation of thyroid hormone and its thyroglobulin protein. Rice bran, which can now be "stabilized," especially from brown rice, remains a rich, important and valuable source of B1 and other B vitamins. Other food sources of thiamine include oatmeal, sunflower seeds, flax seeds, whole grain rye, asparagus, kale, cauliflower, potatoes, oranges, and eggs.

Riboflavin: 100 mg

Riboflavin, also known as vitamin B2, is an essential ingredient in thyroid regulation. Riboflavin has been clinically shown to assist in the production of the primary thyroid hormone, T4. Through its role in the electron transport chain, riboflavin is also a factor in metabolism and energy production, both under the purview of the thyroid. Riboflavin is found in milk, almonds, eggs, spinach and chicken. There is no known toxicity, even at a high dose like this. Antidepressants tend to deplete riboflavin from the body making supplementation necessary.

Magnesium: 200 mg

Low magnesium levels have long been associated with low thyroid function. Magnesium supports thyroid hormone activity and helps regulate thyroid function. Our Standard American Diet (SAD), high in processed food, is the primary cause of magnesium deficiency, which affects at least 7 of 10 Americans. Magnesium is an important element in the production of calcitonin, an essential substance that reduces calcium levels in the blood. People with hyperthyroidism (too high thyroid function) are often magnesium deficient and magnesium supplementation can relieve their symptoms.

Foods that are rich in magnesium include meats, nuts and seeds, garbanzo beans, molasses, legumes, dairy products and some whole grains, including oats and rice. Green leafy vegetables are also a good source of magnesium.

Manganese: 10 mg

Manganese is essential for proper thyroid hormone metabolism. Manganese is an essential trace mineral, meaning that it is vital for body function but only small amounts are needed. Manganese is linked to thyroid function in a rather convoluted way by helping balance through the neurotransmitter dopamine, another factor in proper thyroid hormone function. Excessive amounts of manganese can cause hyperthyroidism. Manganese is found in nuts, brown rice, garbanzo beans, spinach, pineapple, pumpkin seeds, rye and soybeans.

Vitamin C: 1200 mg

Hormone actions, including thyroid hormone production, are dependent on adequate vitamin C levels. Tyrosinase, a part of the vitamin C molecule, activates copper, allowing it to function in stimulating energy metabolism and thyroid hormone production. Vitamin C is found in virtually all fruits and berries, tomatoes, green peppers, dark green leafy vegetables and broccoli. The best source of C: Eat an orange every day in winter and loads of berries and fresh fruit in the warmer months.

AUTHOR'S CHOICE

I recommend a triple iodine compound to my patients because I have found it to be the most effective in raising iodine to optimal levels, neutralizing bromine toxicity, protecting the thyroid, improving thyroid function and preserving breast and prostate health.

Terry Naturally Tri-Iodine is the only brand that contains all three forms of essential iodine: potassium iodide, sodium iodide and molecular iodine.

Terry Naturally Thyroid Care product contains all three forms of iodine plus L-tyrosine for extra thyroid support. I continually try to determine what is needed and which products are best and most important for maintaining optimal long term health.

I can also heartily recommend Terry Naturally's excellent product, Iodine Co-Factors, which contains all the vitamins and minerals found in the list on pages 71–73.

I have found these products to be of the highest quality and I am convinced they provide my patients with the tools to optimize iodine sufficiency throughout the body.

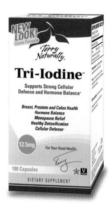 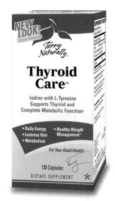 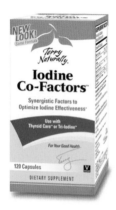

Iodophobia

Drs. Abraham and Brownstein have created a tongue-in-cheek psychological condition called "medical iodophobia" or doctors' fear of iodine.

Many doctors suffer from it, they quip:

"A new syndrome, medical iodophobia, was recently reported with symptoms of split personality, double standards, amnesia, confusion and altered state of consciousness. Medical iodophobia has reached pandemic proportion and it is highly contagious (iatrogenic iodophobia). A century ago, non-radioactive forms of inorganic iodine were considered a panacea for all human ills, but today, they are avoided by physicians like leprosy. We have previously discussed the factors involved in this medical iodophobia. If iodine deficiency is the cause of medical iodophobia, this syndrome would become self-perpetuating. Unfortunately, physicians are afraid of the element that is, most likely, the cure of their phobia."

Fortunately, there are progressive physicians who continue to explore new ways to use this miraculous mineral for an ever-increasing number of diseases beyond thyroid disorders. Their ability to heal and prevent various illnesses using this time-tested mineral is gaining the attention of people all over the world, and interest is growing in creating clinically validated protocols featuring medicinal iodine.

Further research regarding the toxic effects of bromine and the other halogens cannot come fast enough, but the evidence as presented in this text and the previously mentioned texts of the above authors is beyond compelling. It is hard to understand why it is not more widely recognized.

Resources

Books

Thompson, Robert and Barnes, Kathleen, *The Calcium Lie 2: What Your Doctor Still Doesn't Know* (Take Charge Books, 2013).

Brownstein, David, M.D. *Iodine: Why You Need it, Why You Can't Live Without It* (Medical Alternatives Press, 2009).

Brownstein, David, M.D. *Overcoming Thyroid Disorders*, Third Edition (Medical Alternatives Press, 2008).

Walsh, William, *Nutrient Power: Heal Your Biochemistry and Heal Your Brain* (Sky Horse Publishing, 2014).

Websites

http://www.calciumlie.com

http://iodineonmymind.com

http://theiodineproject.webs.com/

http://www.iccidd.org

http://www.cancerchoices.org

http://www.terrytalksnutrition.com

http://STTM.com

Scientific References

Chapter 1: We All Need It and Most of Us Don't Get Enough

Pearce EN, Andersson M et al. Global Iodine Nutrition: Where do we stand in 2013? *Thyroid*. 2013 May;23(5):523–8. doi: 10.1089/thy.2013.0128. Epub 2013 Apr 18.

Caldwell KL, Jones R, Hollowell JG. Urinary iodine concentration: United States National Health And Nutrition Examination Survey 2001–2002. *Thyroid*. Jul 2005;15(7):692–9.

Caldwell, KL, Miller GA et al. Iodine status of the U.S. population, National Health and Nutrition Examination Survey 2003–2004. Thyroid 2008 Nov;18(11): 1207–14. doi: 10.1089/thy.2008.0161.

Hollowell JG, Staehling NW et al. Iodine nutrition in the United States. Trends and public health implications: iodine excretion data from National Health and Nutrition Examination Surveys I and III (1971–1974 and 1988–1994). *J Clin Endocrinol Metab*. Oct 1998;83(10):3401–8.

Abraham, GE, Flechas, J.D. et al. Orthoiodosupplementation: Iodine Sufficiency Of The Whole Human Body. *The Original Internist* 2002 9:30–41.

Abraham, GE. The historical background of the iodine project. *The Original Internist* 2005 12(2):57–66.

Chapter 2: When Things Go Wrong

Hollowell JG, Staehling NW et al. Iodine nutrition in the United States. Trends and public health implications: iodine excretion data from National Health and Nutrition Examination Surveys I and III (1971–1974 and 1988–1994) *J Clin Endo Metab* Oct;83(10):3401–8.

Levothyroxine sales: Top 100 Selling Drugs of 2013. Available at: http://www.medscape.com/viewarticle/820011. Accessed on June 16, 2014.

Eskin BA. Iodine and mammary cancer. *J Trace Elem Med Biol.* 2013 Oct;27(4): 302–6. doi: 10.1016/j.jtemb.2013.07.002. Epub 2013 Jul 16.

Zimmerman MB. The role of iodine in human growth and development. *Med Hypotheses.* 1987 Nov;24(3):249–63.

Foster HD. Disease family trees: the possible roles of iodine in goitre, cretinism, multiple sclerosis, amyotrophic lateral sclerosis, Alzheimer's and Parkinson's diseases and cancers of the thyroid, nervous system and skin. *Nutr Hosp.* 2012 Sep-Oct;27(5):1610–8. doi: 10.3305/nh.2012.27.5.5931.

Northen, C. U.S. Senate. 1936. Modern Miracle Men, Article by Rex Beach Relating to Proper Food Mineral Balances. 74th Congress, 2nd Session, Serial Set 10016. *U.S. Gov't Printing Office,* Washington, D.C.

Davis D. Changes in USDA Food Composition Data for 43 Garden Crops, 1950 to 1999. *Journal of the American College of Nutrition* Vol. 23, No. 6, 669–682 (2004).

Dasqupta PK, Liu Y et al. Iodine nutrition: iodine content of iodized salt in the United States. *Environ Sci Technol.* 2008 Feb 15;42(4):1315–23.

Vobecky M et al. Interaction of Bromine with Iodine in the Rat Thyroid Gland at Enhanced Bromide Intake. *Biol Trace Elem Res* 1996.

Messina M, Redmond G. Effects of soy protein and soybean isoflavones on thyroid function in healthy adults and hypothyroid patients: a review of the relevant literature. *Thyroid.* 2006 Mar;16(3):249–58.

Bell DS, Ovalle F. Use of soy protein supplement and resultant need for increased dose of levothyroxine. *Endocr Pract.* 2001 May-Jun;7(3):193–4.

Bull RJ, Birnbaum L et al. Water Chlorination: Essential Process or Cancer Hazard? *Toxicol. Sci.* (1995) 28 (2): 155–166. doi: 10.1093/toxsci/28.2.155.

Abraham, G.E., Brownstein, D. Validation of the orthoiodosupplementation program: A Rebuttal of Dr. Gaby's Editorial on iodine. *The Original Internist* 12(4): 184–194, 20.

Chapter 3: Iodine, Thyroid Disorders, Obesity and More

Al-Attas OS, Al-DSaghri NM et al. Urinary iodine is associated with insulin resistance in subjects with diabetes mellitus type 2. *Exp Clin Endocrinol Diabetes.* 2012 Nov;120(10):618–22. doi: 10.1055/s-0032–1323816. Epub 2012 Nov 30.

Schneider DF, Nookala R. Thyroidectomy as Primary Treatment Optimizes Body Mass Index in Patients with Hyperthyroidism. *Ann Surg Oncol.* 2014 Feb 13. [Epub ahead of print]

Cancer Res 1979;39:729–734.

Cave WT, Dunn JT et al. Thyroidectomy as Primary Treatment Optimizes Body Mass Index in Patients with Hyperthyroidism.

Ann Surg Oncol. 2014 Feb 13. [Epub ahead of print]

Chapter 4: Iodine, Women and Breast Health

Ghent WR, Eskin BA. Iodine replacement in fibrocystic disease of the breast. *Can J Surg.* 1993 Oct;36(5):453–60.

Krouse TB et al., Age-Related Changes Resembling Fibrocystic Disease in Iodine-Blocked Rat Breasts, *Arch Pathol Lab Med.* 1979 Nov;103(12):631–4.

Cann SA., et al., Hypothesis: Iodine, Selenium, and the Development of Breast Cancer. *Cancer Causes Control.* 2000 Feb;11(2):121–7.

Siiteri PK, Sholtz RI, Cirillo PM, et al. Prospective study of estrogens during pregnancy and risk of breast cancer. Public Health Institute, Berkeley, CA. [Findings presented at Dept of Defense Breast Cancer Research Meeting] 2002 Sept. 26.

Stoddard FR, Brooks Ad et al. Iodine Alters Gene Expression in the MCF7 Breast Cancer Cell Line: Evidence for an Anti-Estrogen Effect of Iodine. *Int J Med Sci* 2008; 5(4):189–196. doi:10.7150/ijms.5.189.

Eskin BA. Iodine and breast cancer A 1982 update. *Biol Trace Elem Res.* 1983 Aug;5(4–5):399–412. doi: 10.1007/BF02987224.

Eskin BA, Sparks CE et al. The intracellular metabolism of iodine in carcinogenesis. *Biol Trace Elem Res.* 1979 Jun;1(2):101–17. doi: 10.1007/BF02821706.

Nathanson L. In vivo prediction of drug sensitivity with cancer-seeking isotopes. *Natl Cancer Inst Monogr.* 1971 Dec;34:225–33.

Chapter 5: Iodine and Other Forms of Cancer

Xhaard C, Ren Y et al. Differentiated thyroid carcinoma risk factors in French Polynesia. *Asian Pac J Cancer Prev.* 2014;15(6):2675–80.

Stocks P. Cancer and goiter. *Biometrika* 16:364–401 1924

Venturi S, Donati FM et al. Role of iodine in evolution and carcinogenesis of thyroid, breast and stomach. *Adv Clin Path.* 2000 Jan;4(1):11–7.

Davies L, Welch HG. Current thyroid cancer trends in the United States. *JAMA Otolaryngol Head Neck Surg.* 2014 Apr;140(4):317–22).

Abnet CC, Fan J F et al. Self-reported goiter is associated with a significantly increased risk of gastric non-cardiac adenocarcinoma in a large population-based Chinese cohort. *Int J Cancer* 2006 119:1508–1510.

Smith JJ et al. Cancer after thyroidectomy: a multi-institutional experience with 1,523 patients. *J Am Coll Surg* 2013;216:571–9. Epub February 8, 2013.

Zhang L and others. Nonradioactive iodide effectively induces apoptosis in genetically modified lung cancer cells. *Cancer Res* 2003;63:5065–5072.

Chapter 6: Iodine and Children

Women of reproductive age have low iodine levels:

CDC's Second Nutrition Report: a comprehensive biochemical assessment of the nutrition status of the US population. Available at: http://www.cdc.gov/nutritionreport/pdf/4Page_%202nd%20Nutrition%20Report_508_032912.pdf. Accessed on June 16, 2014).

Recommendation for iodine supplementation in pregnant and breastfeeding women:

Council on Environmental Health. Iodine deficiency, pollutant chemicals, and the thyroid: new information on an old problem. *Pediatrics.* 2014 May 26. pii: peds. 2014–0900.

Leung AM, Brent GA. Children of mothers with iodine deficiency during pregnancy are more likely to have lower verbal IQ and reading scores at 8–9 years of age. *Evid Based Nurs.* 2013 Dec 12. doi: 10.1136/eb-2013–101585. [Epub ahead of print]

Rayman M et al. Maternal iodine deficiency may threaten children's IQ. *BMJ.* 2013 May 28;346:f3400. doi: 10.1136/bmj.f3400.

Hamza RT, Hewedi Dh et al. et al. Iodine deficiency in Egyptian autistic children and their mothers: relation to disease severity. *Arch Med Res.* 2013 Oct;44(7): 555–61.doi: 0.1016/j.arcmed.2013.09.012. Epub 2013 Oct 10.

Roman GC, Ghassabian A et al. Association of gestational maternal hypothyroxinemia and increased autism risk. *Ann Neurol.* 2013 Nov;74(5):733–42. doi: 10.1002/ana.23976. Epub 2013 Aug 13.

Hetzel BS. Iodine and neuropsychological development. *J Nutr.* 2000;130(2S Suppl):493S–495S.

Tiwari BD, Godbole MM et al. Learning disabilities and poor motivation to achieve due to prolonged iodine deficiency. *Am J Clin Nutr.* 1996;63(5):782–786.

Bleichrodt N, Shrestha RM, West CE, Hautvast JG, van de Vijver FJ, Born MP. The benefits of adequate iodine intake. *Nutr Rev.* 1996;54(4 Pt 2):S72–78.

Bath SC, Steer CD, Golding J, Emmett P, Rayman MP. Effect of inadequate iodine status in UK pregnant women on cognitive outcomes in their children: results from the Avon Longitudinal Study of Parents and Children (ALSPAC). *Lancet.* Jul 27 2013;382(9889):331–7.

Santiago-Fernandez P, Torres-Barahona R, Muela-Martínez JA, et al. Intelligence quotient and iodine intake: a cross-sectional study in children. *J Clin Endocrinol Metab.* Aug 2004;89(8):3851–7.

Chapter 7: Iodine, Detoxification and Other Health Conditions

Distiller LA, Polakow ES et al. Type 2 diabetes mellitus and hypothyroidism: the possible influence of metformin therapy. *Diabet Med.* 2014 Feb;31(2):172–5. doi: 10.1111/dme.12342. Epub 2013 Nov 18.

Al-Attas OS, Al-Daghri NM et al. Urinary iodine is associated with insulin resistance in subjects with diabetes mellitus type 2. *Exp Clin Endocrinol Diabetes.* 2012 Nov;120(10):618–22. doi: 10.1055/s-0032–1323816. Epub 2012 Nov 30.

Asranna A, Taneja RS et al. Dyslipidemia in subclinical hypothyroidism and the effect of thyroxine on lipid profile. *Indian J Endocrinol Metab.* 2012 Dec;16(Suppl 2):S347–9. doi: 10.4103/2230–8210.104086.

Flechas J. The potential of oxytocin, nitric oxide, and iodine. *Altern Ther Health Med.* 2013 Jul-Aug;19(4):50–6.

Lowe, John et al. Thyroid Status of Fibromyalgia patients. *Myofascial Therapy,* 3(1): 47–53. 1998.

Valentino R, Savastano S et al. Screening a coastal population in Southern Italy: iodine deficiency and prevalence of goitre: nutritional aspects and cardiovascular risk factors. *Nutr Metab Cardiovasc Dis.* 2004 Feb;14(1):15–9.

Hoption Cann SA. Hypothesis: dietary iodine intake in the etiology of cardiovascular disease. *J Am Coll Nutr.* 2006 Feb;25(1):1–11.

Stone OJ. The role of the primitive sea in the natural selection of iodides as a regulating factor in inflammation. *Med Hypotheses.* 1988 25:125–129

Foster HD. Disease family trees: the possible roles of iodine in goitre, cretinism, multiple sclerosis, amyotrophic lateral sclerosis, Alzheimer's and Parkinson's diseases and cancers of the thyroid, nervous system and skin. *Med Hypotheses.* 1987 Nov;24(3):249–63.

Zimmermann MB, Jooste PL, Pandav CS. Iodine-deficiency disorders. *Lancet.* Oct 4 2008;372(9645):1251–62.

Chapter 8: The Right Iodine

Abraham, GE, Handal RC et al. A Simplified Procedure for the Measurement of Urine Iodide Levels by the Ion-Selective Electrode Assay in a Clinical Setting. *The Original Internist* Vol 13, No. 3, 125–135, September 2006.

Abraham, GE, The historical background of the iodine project. *The Original Internist* 12(2):57–66, 2005.

Abraham, GE. The History of Iodine in Medicine Part III: Thyroid Fixation and Medical Iodophobia. *The Original Internist,* 2006;13: 71–78.

Abraham, GE. The safe and effective implementation of orthoiodosupplementation in medical practice. *The Original Internist,* 2004;11:17–36.

About the Author

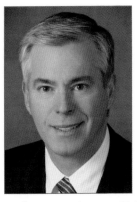

Dr. Robert Thompson currently practices integrative, anti-aging, and holistic medicine in Soldotna and Anchorage, Alaska.

He is a board certified OB/Gyn by training at Pennsylvania State University where he served as chief resident and clinical instructor. He is a fellow of the American College of Obstetrics and Gynecology. He practiced OB/GYN for over 30 years, but now limits his practice to integrative and preventive medicine and bio-identical hormone replacement therapy.

Dr. Thompson was chosen by his peers to be in the top 5% of physicians in the USA, as Best Physicians in America in 1996.

He is considered an authority on hypothyroidism diagnosis and treatment and bio-identical hormone replacement therapy for both men and women. He has developed and perfected bio-identical trans mucosal hormone replacement (TMRx), leading the world in this method of bio-identical hormone replacement.

He is an expert and authority in the clinical application of hair tissue mineral analysis (HTMA) in nutrition and disease.

Dr. Thompson discovered and published an original theory on

the principle of mineral substitution in human physiology, 2013, called the Thompson-Doberiner Theory. He discovered and published the first accurate report on Type 2 Hypothyroidism, its clinical cause and correct method of diagnosis. He described it accurately for the first time in 2008 in *The Calcium Lie: What Your Doctor Doesn't Know Might Kill You* (1st edition).

He also organized hypothyroidism into six reproducible and specifically treatable types in 2013 which is actually based on existing clinical research and scientific literature, in *The Calcium Lie 2: What Your Doctor Still Doesn't Know* (Take Charge Books, 2013).

Dr. Thompson lives in Soldotna, Alaska, where he enjoys the outdoors and the peace and beauty of Alaska's wilderness, living on the edge of the Kenai National Wildlife Refuge.

He sees moose almost daily, caribou not infrequently, grizzly bears, too often (and yes he is packing a gun in the summer, even in the neighborhood), black bears, eagles, cranes, swans, loons, and more.

Dr. Thompson is a concert violinist and performs regularly for charity fund raisers. He serves as president of the board of directors of Love INC of the Kenai Peninsula, a ministry caring for the poor and he is secretary of the board for the Kenai Peninsula Orchestra for whom he plays first violin.

He loves cooking, art and music. He canoes, floats rivers, fishes, hunts, skis cross country and downhill, ski jours, trains and raises his four Labrador retrievers. He often jokes that he lives in a dog house! He snow machines, water skis, helps build houses year round, and is a teaching assistant for 5th and 6th grade Sunday School.

He has two grown children, Tiffany, a Neonatal Intensive Care Charge Nurse, and Nate, a professional hockey player for the Anaheim Ducks.

He served as a lieutenant colonel in the United States Army Reserves Medical Corps with distinction. He received an honorable discharge in June 2011.